MW01491016

W. EUGENE KNOX

Control Processes
in Neoplasia

Symposia on Metabolic Regulation

Editors

Myron A. Mehlman   Richard W. Hanson

Energy Metabolism and the Regulation of Metabolic Processes in Mitochondria, 1972

The Role of Membranes in Metabolic Regulation, 1972

Control Processes in Neoplasia, 1973

ACADEMIC PRESS RAPID MANUSCRIPT REPRODUCTION

Control Processes in Neoplasia

Edited by

Myron A. Mehlman

Department of Biochemistry
University of Nebraska College of Medicine
Omaha, Nebraska

Richard W. Hanson

Fels Research Institute and Department
of Biochemistry
Temple University Medical School
Philadelphia, Pennsylvania

Proceedings of a Symposium held at the
University of Nebraska Medical Center
Omaha, Nebraska, June 11-12, 1973

Academic Press, Inc.   New York and London   1974
A Subsidiary of Harcourt Brace Jovanovich, Publishers

ACADEMIC PRESS, INC.
111 Fifth Avenue, New York, New York 10003

United Kingdom Edition published by
ACADEMIC PRESS, INC. (LONDON) LTD.
24/28 Oval Road. London NW1

Library of Congress Cataloging in Publication Data
Main entry under title:

Control processes in neoplasia.

        (Symposia on metabolic regulation)
        1.   Carcinogenesis–Congresses.   2.   Metabolic regu-
lation–Congresses.   3.   Cellular control mechanisms–
Congress.   I.   Mehlman, Myron A., ed.   II.   Hanson,
Richard W., ed.   III.   Series.   [DNLM: 1.   Neoplasms–
Metabolism–Congresses.   QZ200 C764 1973]
RC261.C735   616.9'94'071   73–21861
ISBN 0–12–487860–1

CONTENTS

CONTENTS

CONTRIBUTORS

Ernest Borek, Department of Microbiology, University of Colorado Medical Center, Denver, Colorado 80220

Thaddeus Borun, Fels Research Institute, Temple University School of Medicine, Philadelphia, Pennsylvania 19140

Richard Carchman, Laboratory of Molecular Biology, National Cancer Institute, National Institutes of Health, Bethesda, Maryland 20014

Emmanuel Farber, Fels Research Institute, Temple University School of Medicine, Philadelphia, Pennsylvania 19140

James N. Ihle, Carcinogenesis Program, Biology Division, Oak Ridge National Laboratory, Oak Ridge, Tennessee 37830

Francis Kenney, Carcinogenesis Program, Biology Division, Oak Ridge National Laboratory, Oak Ridge, Tennessee 37830

Sylvia Kerr, Department of Surgery, University of Colorado Medical Center, Denver, Colorado 80220

Saul Kit, Division of Biochemical Virology, Baylor University College of Medicine, Houston, Texas 77025

Eugene Knox, Department of Biological Chemistry, Harvard Medical School and the Cancer Research Institute, New England Deaconess Hospital, Boston, Massachusetts 02215

Kai-Lin Lee, Carcinogenesis Program, Biology Division, Oak Ridge National Laboratory, Oak Ridge, Tennessee 37830

Wai-Choi Leung, Division of Biochemical Virology, Baylor University College of Medicine, Houston, Texas 77025

Dawn Marks, Fels Research Institute, Temple University School of Medicine, Philadelphia, Pennsylvania 19140

Woon Ki Paik, Fels Research Institute, Temple University School of Medicine, Philadelphia, Pennsylvania 19140

D. S. R. Sarma, Fels Research Institute, Temple University School of Medicine, Philadelphia, Pennsylvania 19140

Gordon Tomkins, University of California, San Francisco, San Francisco, California 94143

David Trkula, Division of Biochemical Virology, Baylor University College of Medicine, Houston, Texas 77025

Sidney Weinhouse, Fels Research Institute and the Department of Biochemistry, Temple University School of Medicine, Philadelphia, Pennsylvania 19140

PREFACE

Metabolic regulation is a highly diversified field encompassing a wide range of disciplines. This yearly symposium, held at the University of Nebraska School of Medicine in Omaha, is aimed at bringing together scientists in specific areas of metabolic regulation to discuss recent advances in the field. This book, the third in the series, is the result of a meeting held on June 11-12, 1973, and deals with alterations in metabolic regulation associated with neoplasia. The meeting was divided into three major sections involving control processes at the level of DNA (transcriptional events) of RNA (translational and associated events) and on the broad effects that alterations in these processes may have on enzymes in neoplastic tissues. We attempted, in selecting participants in this symposium, to include scientists with well established reputations in this area as well as younger investigators whose work shows promise of providing new and interesting directions for future advances. We have also imposed no restrictions on the authors concerning the style, scope or method of presentation of their chapters, so that the responsibility for the scientific content of each chapter is theirs.

This volume is dedicated to Professor Sidney Weinhouse in his sixty-fifth year, in honor of his long and distinguished career in two areas, metabolic regulation and the biochemical basis of neoplasia. Sidney Weinhouse worked in cancer research when most biochemists found the area unfashionable. That it now represents a major field of biochemical experimentation is, in no small part, due to his efforts.

We are indebted to Dr. Emmanuel Farber for his invaluable assistance in organizing this symposium. We also wish to thank Miss Rita Daly and the Center for Continuing Education at the University of Nebraska Medical Center for their excellent work in coordinating the many details required to make a meeting of this type a success. Finally, we thank Dr. Philippe Shubik, of The Eppley Institute for Research in Cancer, for making available to us facilities of his Institute for our symposium.

Myron A. Mehlman
Richard W. Hanson

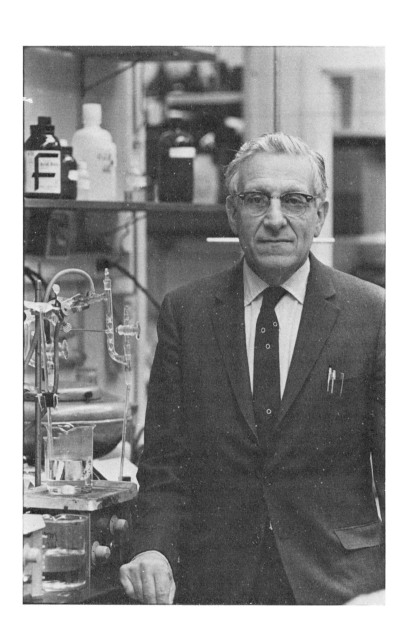

DEDICATION

Relevancy in science is now the by-word and many biologists find them-selves deeply involved in attempting to apply basic findings to problems dealing with disease. Despite the great advances made in understanding the etiology of the major human diseases—cancer, heart disease, diabetes—they continue to take their toll in death and suffering. For scientists they are a challenge to our fundamental belief that in understanding the basic mecha-nisms of normal cell function we can provide a rational basis for an approach to their cure. The current interest in the mechanisms of neoplasia is built on a broad base of research centered on the molecular alterations which occur in cancer cells. This volume is dedicated to Sidney Weinhouse, who has been one of the outstanding figures in this area. Before it was fashionable for bio-chemists to work on cancer, before relevancy was the trend, he was deeply involved in biochemical studies with tumors.

Dr. Weinhouse began his scientific studies at a time when biochemistry was coming into prominence. He was among the first to use radio-isotopes in metabolic studies and his initial work was instrumental in establishing the pathway of ketone body formation in the liver. This work confirmed the β-oxidation hypothesis proposed in 1904 by Knoop and provided a model for later studies using isotopes of carbon. Having received his Ph.D. in organic chemistry from the University of Chicago in 1936, he was well prepared for work which required the synthesis of each of the radioactive substrates used in these experiments. He moved to the Institute for Cancer Research in Philadelphia in 1950, where he began a detailed study of the metabolism of carbohydrates, lipids and amino acids in both normal and cancer tissue. This work is well known and widely cited, and extends into areas as diverse as ketone body metabolism in diabetes, the metabolic effects of insulin as well as studies with tumor tissues. Together with David DiPietro, he first recog-nized the existence of a liver enzyme with a high K_m for glucose. The discovery of glucokinase was a major advance in carbohydrate metabolism since this enzyme regulates the rate of uptake of glucose by the liver.

Weinhouse's firm grounding in biochemistry has always been his greatest asset in the cancer field. The interplay between glycolysis and respiration in cancer tissue was considered to be a fundamental aspect of neoplasia. Warburg had suggested in 1930 that cancer originates when a normal cell adapts to anerobic metabolism as a means of survival after injury to its respiratory system. This concept was challenged by Weinhouse in a short article in *Science* (**124**: 267, 1956) entitled "On Respiratory Impairment in Cancer Cells". In criticizing this theory, he reviewed some of the earlier data used by Warburg in support of his concept: "... in Table 1, he [Warburg] shows that whereas liver, kidney and embryo have Q_{O_2}'s of –15, the ascites tumor has a Q_{O_2} of –7. On these grounds he concludes that the tumor cannot utilize sufficient oxygen for its needs and thus requires fermentative energy. On the assumption that each mole of lactic acid formed from glucose yields 1 mole of ATP and each mole of oxygen consumed gives rise to 7 moles of ATP, he calculates that the tumor obtains more than half of its potential phosphate bond energy by glycolysis whereas the three noncancer tissues obtain theirs mainly by respiration. Accepting these results at their face value, it is still necessary to ask why some normal tissues manage to survive without glycolysis with Q_{O_2}'s of –3 to –6; also why some tumors glycolyze highly with Q_{O_2}'s as high as –10 to –20? It is also pertinent to ask why certain nonneoplastic tissues, with moderate to high oxygen uptake—for example, brain, retina, kidney, medulla and intestinal mucosa—glycolyze as highly as many tumors? It is evident that all tumors produce large amounts of lactic acid, but so do many noncancer tissues; and just as noncancer tissues display a wide diversity in oxygen uptake, so do tumors." This brief article along with the replies by Warburg and by Burk make fascinating reading today, 18 years after they were published. Support for Weinhouse's point of view grew steadily and we now recognize that altered respiration and glycolysis are not essential biochemical lesions in neoplastic transformation.

In 1963, Sidney Weinhouse became the director of the Fels Research Institute at Temple University and in 1969 was appointed editor of *Cancer Research.* He has distinguished himself in both capacities. As editor of *Cancer Research* he has worked to improve the journal, to up-grade its scientific content and at the same time preserve its relevance to investigators more directly involved with the clinical aspects of cancer. Those of us who have been privileged to work with him at the Fels Research Institute, owe this unusual man our lasting gratitude. He has shown us how to work together in a spirit of common good-will in a laboratory where scientists can disagree without disrespect and can praise without flattering. He is one of those rare individuals who by their presence bring honor and prestige to a university. Now in his sixty-fifth year, and approaching retirement from his duties as department chairman, he continues actively to pursue his research into the relationship between isoenzymes and neoplasia. This volume on control processes in neoplasia is fittingly dedicated to Sidney Weinhouse in appreciation of his pioneering research in this area, with our thanks and appreciation.

Richard W. Hanson
Philadelphia, 1973

ISOZYME ALTERATIONS AND METABOLISM OF EXPERIMENTAL LIVER NEOPLASMS

Sidney Weinhouse

Introduction

Ever since the modern era of biochemical research in cancer began, with the epoch-making work of Otto Warburg some 50 years ago, biochemists have been seeking the philosopher's stone of cancer--a unique characteristic that would provide a target for the selective destruction of the cancer cell; and that would reveal the molecular basis for the neoplastic transformation. Unfortunately, neither objective has been reached. Although the history of cancer biochemistry has many notable discoveries to its credit, it is becoming ever more clear that the complexities of cellular regulation confound any simplistic solution to the mystery of neoplasia. However, progress has been made, even if such progress may represent only the correction of past errors. In this presentation I would like to emphasize two areas in which some modicum of progress can be recorded. One concerns the conception of cancer as a disorder or aberration of normal differentiation; the second, not entirely unrelated to the first, concerns the significance of the high aerobic glycolysis to the neoplastic process.

A common thread, interwoven through much of the recent literature, is that cancer is associated with aberrant mechanisms of gene expresssion, manifested by the appearance of proteins inappropriate to the cell of origin. The clinical literature abounds with examples of the ectopic production of polypeptide hormones in nonendocrine tumors (1-4). According to the immunologic literature, proteins identifiable as antigens in normal, adult differentiated tissues are lost in tumors, while neo-antigens appear that are absent from the cell of origin but may be present in fetal tissue (5-12). This recurring pattern suggests that genes coding for fetal proteins, which have been inactivated during normal embryonic development, become reactivated in cancer. In recent years,

1

work from our own and other laboratories has resulted in
strikingly similar findings with regard to enzymes (13-18).
In the time available I would like to describe these results,
and to discuss with you their significance to the metabolic
behavior of neoplastic cells.

Methods and Results

The Morris Hepatomas

Before proceeding, however, I should describe our experimental system which comprises a series of chemically-
induced transplantable liver neoplasms of the rat known as
the Morris Hepatomas (19-21). The availability of this
spectrum of parenchymal cell neoplasms provides a unique
opportunity for exploring molecular parameters of neoplasia.
As shown in Table 1, they may conveniently be divided into
three classes on the basis of their degree of differentiation
as judged by usual histologic criteria. The highly differentiated tumors, of which there are relatively few examples,
grow very slowly. The growth rate, which can be assessed
from the average time between transplantation, ranges from
3 to 4 months up to well over a year. The many well-differentiated Morris hepatomas grow somewhat more rapidly, taking
from 2 to 6 months for a transplant generation; and the poorly
differentiated tumors grow so rapidly as to kill their hosts
in less than 1 month down to about 10 days. The highly-
differentiated tumors have the normal liver chromosome number and karyotype, the well-differentiated differ slightly,
and the poorly differentiated deviate markedly in chromosome
karyotype and number, from those of rat liver. Respiration
decreases moderately with loss of differentiation, but the
most striking biochemical feature is the low or negligible
glycolysis in the well-differentiated tumors; this is in
decided contrast with the usual high level of glycolysis in
the poorly differentiated tumors (22-24).
These hepatomas, ranging widely in their growth rate
and in the degree of differentiation, yet originating from
a single cell type, the parenchymal cell of the liver, obviously provide an ideal model system for exploring molecular
mechanisms underlying tumor behavior. Prompted by the wide
range of glycolytic activity exhibited by these hepatomas,
we undertook a study of their enzymology and metabolism directed primarily to learn why they differ in their glycolytic

2

TABLE 1

General Properties of Morris Hepatomas

Property	Degree of Differentiation		
	High	Well	Poor
Growth rate	Very low	Low	Rapid
Chromosome number	Normal	Nearly normal	Abnormal
Chromosome karyotype	Normal	Nearly normal	Abnormal
Respiration	High	Moderate	Moderately low
Glycolysis	Low	Low	High
Enzyme Pattern	Liver-like	Some deletions	Many deletions

3

activity; and secondarily to ascertain to what extent enzymes
playing key roles in hepatic function are lost or retained
in these hepatomas.

Isozyme Alterations

Four enzymes will be discussed, each of which plays a
key role in hepatic carbohydrate metabolism. Each exists in
multiple forms, and in each instance the liver possesses an
isozyme uniquely tailored to important hepatic function
(Table 2). The hepatic type of glucose-ATP phosphotransferase known as glucokinase, is under host control through its
adaptive responsiveness to dietary glucose and insulin; and
its kinetic properties and its high specificity toward glucose make it particularly significant in liver physiology.
It is accompanied by low activities of three other relatively
non-specific hexokinases. The hepatic aldolase, aldolase B,
is essentially the sole form in adult rat liver. It is highly
active toward fructose-1-phosphate, the first product of
cellular metabolism of fructose, and thus has a crucial role
in the utilization of this sugar. The L-type pyruvate kinase,
like glucokinase, is adaptive to diet and insulin, and also
plays a key role in such hepatic functions as glucose utilization and gluconeogenesis. The fourth enzyme, glycogen
phosphorylase, also exists in isozymic forms; in each instance the liver forms have chemical and kinetic properties
that are tailored to the highly regulated processes of glycogen deposition and mobilization.

All four of these enzymes displayed a common pattern of
isozyme alteration, which is described diagrammatically in
Fig. 1 (18,25-27). In normal adult liver, the liver form
is the sole or predominant isozyme, while non-hepatic isozymes are either low or absent in activity. In all instances,
the slow growing, highly differentiated hepatomas exhibited
a similar pattern, with virtually complete retention of the
liver-type isozyme. As dedifferentiation proceeds, and
growth rate increases, the hepatomas lose the liver-type
isozyme activity and isozymes appear that are normally low
or undetectable in the adult liver. With progressive dedifferentiation to the poorly differentiated state, there is
not only a complete or nearly complete disappearance of the
liver type isozyme; there is a replacement by a non-hepatic
type isozyme, sometimes in extremely high activity compared
with the original total enzyme activity in liver. It is
notable that in every instance, the isozyme patterns of the

4

TABLE 2

Enzymes Studied in Rat Liver and Hepatomas

1. Glucose–ATP Phosphotransferases
   Glucose + ATP $\longrightarrow$ Glucose-6-Phosphate + ADP

2. Aldolases
   Fructose-1,6-Diphosphate $\rightleftharpoons$ Glyceraldehyde-3-P + Dihydroxyacetone-P
   Fructose-1-Phosphate $\rightleftharpoons$ Glyceraldehyde + Dihydroxyacetone-P

3. Pyruvate Kinases
   Phosphoenolpyruvate + ADP $\longrightarrow$ Pyruvate + ATP

4. Glycogen Phosphorylases
   n Glucose-1-phosphate $\rightleftharpoons$ Glycogen + n Pi

5

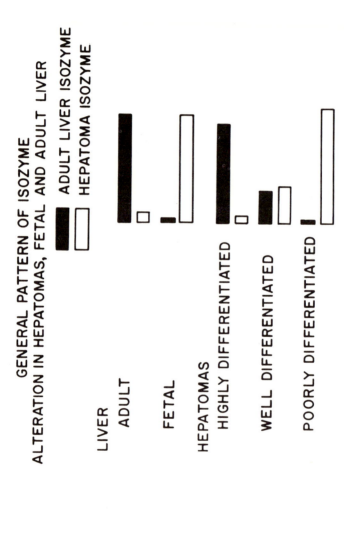

Fig. 1. *Pattern of isozyme alterations in liver and liver neoplasms.* Data presented in diagrammatic form are based on assays of glucose–ATP phosphotransferases, aldolases, pyruvate kinases and glycogen phosphorylases from references cited in the text.

6

poorly differentiated hepatomas resemble those of fetal
liver, where like the poorly differentiated hepatoma, the
adult isozyme activity is low or absent.

Glycogen Phosphorylase

Now I would like to examine these data for two enzymes
in greater detail (Fig. 2). Glycogen phosphorylase isozymes
can be distinguished readily by isoelectric focussing (25–
27). In the top panel is shown the focussing pattern for
skeletal muscle phosphorylase. There is a sharp peak at pH
6.2; and this isozyme is largely in the b form as shown by
the high activity with AMP, designated with open circles,
compared with the low activity without AMP outlined by the
shaded circles. The liver isozyme shown in the second panel,
focusses at pH 5.9, and is further distinguished from the
muscle isozyme in requiring 0.5 M sulfate for full activation,
as outlined by the triangles, even in the presence of AMP
shown in the open circles. In contrast the poorly differentiated Novikoff hepatoma isozyme, which exemplifies other
poorly differentiated hepatomas, has one major peak at pH
5.6, and also differs from the liver isozyme in not requiring
sulfate for activation. The fourth panel shows that a well-
differentiated hepatoma 20 has the liver isozyme as a major
peak, but is also accompanied by a minor hepatoma peak. The
fifth panel shows clearly that in 21-day fetal liver, the
adult liver form is accompanied by a form which focusses like
the hepatoma form. The separate identities of these three
phosphorylase isozymes have been established by immuno-
chemical studies (27) and there appears to be no doubt that
the major or sole isozyme in poorly differentiated hepatomas
is the same as is present in normal fetal liver.

Pyruvate Kinase -- its Role in Aerobic Glycolysis

Another striking example of the same kind is shown
in Fig. 3 (28). Pyruvate kinase is present in adult liver
in a major form, which is tightly held by DEAE-cellulose
and requires a concentration of approximately 0.15 M Cl⁻ ion
for elution. This isozyme has kinetic properties which en-
dow it with unique importance in liver metabolism and is
also responsive to diet and to insulin. It is accompanied
by a low activity of two other isozymes. As shown in the
second panel, the skeletal muscle has a single isozyme which
is less tightly bound and elutes with 0.05 M Cl⁻ ion, and

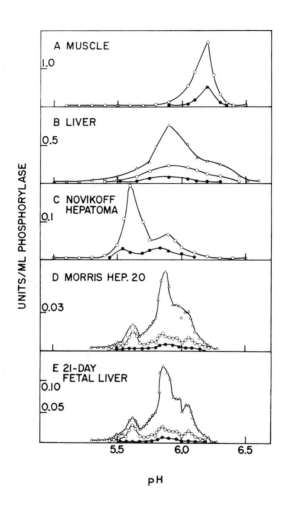

Fig. 2. *Isoelectric focussing patterns of liver and hepatoma glycogen phosphorylases.*

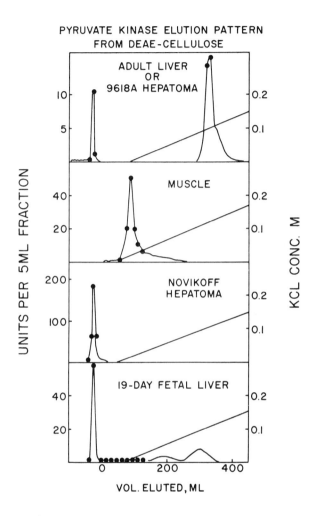

Fig. 3. *Chromatography patterns of pyruvate kinases on DEAE-cellulose obtained on gradient elution with Cl⁻ ion.*

appears to be identical with one of the minor liver forms.
Panel 3 shows that the poorly differentiated Novikoff hepatoma is not held by the resin and is eluted in the void
volume; it appears to be identical with another isozyme
present also in liver at low activity. In the fourth panel
we note that the major tumor isozyme is identical with the
fetal liver form as well--another example of a reactivation
of fetal genes in cancer. I will return to this subject
of fetal manifestations in cancer; but before doing so, I
will digress to discuss the possible significance of this
pattern of pyruvate kinase in cancer metabolism.

In Fig. 4 I have depicted how the isozymes of pyruvate
kinase progress from essentially the liver pattern of high
type L isozyme in the highly differentiated tumors to low
activities in the well-differentiated, to virtual disappearance of the liver isozyme in the poorly differentiated
hepatoma, to be replaced by an extremely high activity of
the hepatoma isozyme.

The extremely high pyruvate kinase activity in the
poorly differentiated tumors prompted up to examine whether
this might provide a clue to the high glycolytic activity
of these hepatomas as well as that of all other poorly-
differentiated tumors. First let us briefly review the
background of the aerobic glycolysis of tumors.

About a half-century ago Otto Warburg, an illustrious
and colorful, indeed a legendary figure in cancer research,
pioneered in what may be called modern cell biology by
applying what were then modern techniques and concepts of
physical chemistry to studies of the cancer cell (29). He
was the first to note that slices of the most diverse tumors
had one common property: they produced large amounts of
lactic acid from glucose. The essence of his experimental
observations, somewhat oversimplified, is shown in Fig. 5.
When normal tissue slices are incubated in a nutrient medium
containing glucose, but in the absence of oxygen, there is
a rapid and continuous utilization of glucose and production
of lactic acid, a process which Warburg termed glycolysis.
However, when the tissues were incubated in oxygen, glycolysis virtually ceased. This decrease of glycolysis brought
about by oxygen was named by Warburg the Pasteur Effect,
after an observation made some 100 years ago by Pasteur
that, when yeast is grown in air, it loses the capability
to ferment glucose to ethanol.

The behavior of tumor slices Warburg found, however,
was quite different. Anaerobic glycolysis was very high;

10

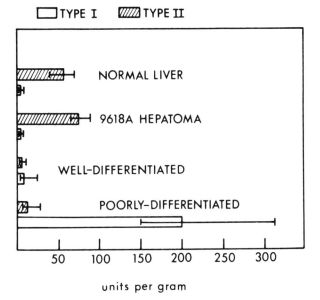

PYRUVATE KINASE ISOZYMES
IN RAT LIVER AND HEPATOMAS

☐ TYPE I   ▨ TYPE II

NORMAL LIVER

9618A HEPATOMA

WELL-DIFFERENTIATED

POORLY-DIFFERENTIATED

50   100   150   200   250   300

units per gram

Fig. 4. *Alteration of pyruvate kinase isozymes in relation to degree of differentiation of hepatic neoplasms.*

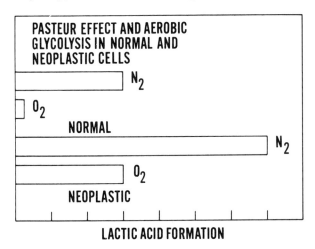

PASTEUR EFFECT AND AEROBIC
GLYCOLYSIS IN NORMAL AND
NEOPLASTIC CELLS

N_2

O_2

NORMAL

N_2

O_2

NEOPLASTIC

LACTIC ACID FORMATION

Fig. 5. *Glycolytic behavior of normal and neoplastic tissues as observed originally by Warburg.*

11

and although a Pasteur Effect was observed, the presence of oxygen did not lead to elimination of glycolysis and aerobic glycolysis remained high. Warburg regarded the persistence of aerobic glycolysis as a key to the neoplastic transformation.

He proposed (Table 3) that the high aerobic glycolysis is the result of a defect in respiration; that cancer results when the cell responds to an irreversible injury to its respiratory mechanism by adopting a fermentative metabolism. According to Warburg, such cells cannot maintain the differentiated state and as undifferentiated cells they grow in uncontrolled fashion. This dictum, vigorously propounded by an illustrious figure in biology, captured the imagination of cancer researchers, and it is difficult to exaggerate the influence of this theory on the direction of cancer research for decades. Moreover, the Pasteur Effect, although still not well understood, has been a focal point for countless studies on metabolism and its regulation.

It was not until about 1950, however, when isotope tracer studies showed that tumors could oxidize glucose to CO_2 at rates comparable with those of normal tissues, that the Warburg hypothesis was seriously questioned (30). Although Warburg defended this theory vigorously, many efforts to discover defects, or even substantive alterations of respiration in cancer, were unsuccessful. A variety of experimental techniques as shown in Table 4 demonstrated that tumors utilize oxygen at low to moderate rates, they contain a full complement of respiratory enzymes and coenzymes, they have mitochondria, which appear normal morphologically and functionally (although they may be low in number in some tumors), the citric acid cycle is operative, and they couple oxidation with ATP production. In the light of our more advanced knowledge of respiration, mitochondrial function, and the interrelationships of the mitochondria with carbohydrate metabolism, the Warburg hypothesis is now regarded at best as a gross oversimplification of exceedingly complex regulatory mechanisms (7,22,31).

In considering enzymatic sites for the Pasteur Effect, an inhibitory effect of respiration on glycolysis, it is logical to consider those enzymes that carry out transfers of phosphate to and from phosphorylated intermediates, since both glycolysis and respiration are intimately coupled to phosphorylation reactions. Much attention has been focussed in recent years on phosphofructokinase because of its remarkable allosteric properties. It is strongly inhib-

12

TABLE 3

The Warburg Hypothesis

---

1. Cancer is initiated by an irreversible injury to respiration.

2. The cancer cell, which survives the injury to respiration, obtains its energy from glycolysis.

3. Such cells cannot maintain the differentiated state; as undifferentiated cells, they grow in uncontrolled fashion.

TABLE 4

Respiratory Characteristics of Tumors

---

1. Utilize oxygen at low to moderate rates.

2. Contain a full complement of respiratory enzymes and coenzymes.

3. Couple respiration with phosphorylation.

4. Mitochondria are normal in structure and function, though may be low in number.

5. Citric acid cycle is operative.

6. Glycolytic and respiratory energy both support biosynthesis.

---

ited by ATP and citrate and is deinhibited by AMP, ADP, and P_i; numerous kinetic experiments point to feedback control on this enzyme by ATP and citrate as the major determinant of glycolytic activity in muscle and possibly also in brain (32,33).

Subsequent transphosphorylation reactions, namely triose phosphate dehydrogenase, where inorganic phosphate is taken up into 1,3-diphosphoglycerate; phosphoglycerate kinase, where phosphate is transferred from 1,3-diphosphoglycerate to ADP to yield 3-phosphoglycerate and ATP; and pyruvate kinase, where phosphate is transferred from phosphoenolpyruvate to ADP to yield pyruvate and ATP are also sites for the Pasteur Effect. These three reactions compete directly for ADP and P_i with the mitochondrial respiratory system, where ADP and P_i are converted to ATP by oxidative phosphorylation coupled with electron transport. They are, therefore, obvious sites for the Pasteur Effect, and indeed this was suggested 30 years ago, independently by Johnson (34) and Lynen (35).

Competition for ADP as a Determinant of Aerobic Glycolysis

Prompted by the extraordinarily high activities of pyruvate kinase in the highly glycolyzing, poorly differentiated hepatomas, we reconsidered this possibility; and we investigated the interactions between glycolytic and respiratory systems of well- and poorly differentiated hepatomas in model systems, with the purpose of measuring the role of pyruvate kinase in determining the relative extents of glycolytic and respiratory ATP production.

To explore the possible role of pyruvate kinase as a determinant of glycolytic rate we designed a model system which is outlined in Fig. 6 (36). A whole, fortified homogenate of liver or hepatoma was incubated in air, with or without fructose diphosphate (FDP) as substrate and with a low, priming concentration of ATP; and O_2 uptake and lactate formation were measured. As outlined in this figure, the formation of lactate from fructose-diphosphate requires a continuous supply of ADP for the two transphosphorylation steps; at phosphoglycerate kinase and at pyruvate kinase. To maintain a steady state, yeast hexokinase and 2-deoxyglucose (2-DG) were added in excess. These additions served several purposes. As rapidly as ATP is formed, whether by glycolytic or respiratory phosphorylation, it is used to

ATP formation during aerobic glycolysis in hepatoma homogenates

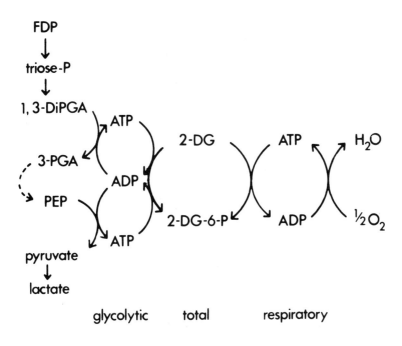

Fig. 6. *Diagram illustrating measurement of glycolytic and respiratory phosphorylation in whole homogenates of liver and hepatomas.*

phosphorylate 2-deoxyglucose. The phosphorylation product
thus formed, namely 2-deoxyglucose-6-phosphate, is inert
and accumulates. Thus, the total ATP production is determined by measuring either 2-DG disappearance or 2DG-6-phos-
phate formation; glycolytic ATP formation is estimated simply as twice the lactate formation; and respiratory phosphorylation is the difference between total and glycolytic
phosphorylation.

Results obtained in this model system are summarized
in Table 5. With liver preparations there is a moderate
increase in total ATP production on addition of FDP, and
no marked change in oxygen uptake. However, without FDP
respiratory phosphorylation was high and glycolytic phosphorylation was negligible. In keeping with the negligible
glycolysis, the addition of FDP increased lactate moderately,
to 9.1, and thereby markedly increased glycolytic phosphorylation to 18.2, largely at the expense of respiratory phosphorylation, which dropped from 19.7 to 7.1 μmoles.

Essentially the same results were obtained with the
well-differentiated, slow growing hepatoma, 5123D. FDP
slightly increased total phosphorylation from 18.3 to 23.7,
had no effect on O_2 uptake, increased lactate only slightly,
and did not diminish respiratory phosphorylation, although
glycolytic phosphorylation was stimulated somewhat. In
contrast the poorly differentiated, rapidly growing 3683
hepatomas responded to FDP addition with greatly increased
total phosphorylation, of which nearly all was glycolytic.

Two important observations were made. First, the
same pattern of low glycolysis in well differentiated hepatomas and high glycolysis in poorly differentiated hepatomas was seen with FDP as substrate as with glucose as
substrate (23). Therefore at least as far as can be inferred from this model system, control of glycolysis is not
at hexokinase or phosphofructokinase, but rather at a step
beyond FDP. Second, the poorly differentiated hepatoma,
with its high activity of pyruvate kinase, competes successfully with its respiratory system for the available ADP;
while the well-differentiated hepatoma, with its low pyruvate kinase activity, has little effect on respiratory ATP
production.

Further evidence for glycolytic control by the glycolytic transphosphorylating enzymes may be seen in Table 6,
in which glycolytic and respiratory systems of well and
poorly differentiated hepatomas were intermixed in the same

model system. With a reconstituted glycolytic supernatant fraction and a particulate respiratory system of the well differentiated 5123 hepatoma, there was a moderate total phosphorylation of 18.6 μmoles, of which nearly all was respiratory. With similarly reconstituted fractions of the poorly differentiated hepatoma 3683, there was a very high total phosphorylation, of which practically all was glycolytic phosphorylation. By intermixing the low glycolyzing supernatant of the well differentiated hepatoma with the respiratory particles of the poorly differentiated hepatoma, we see that the normally low glycolyzing 5123 supernatant becomes high glycolyzing when freed from the competition with its more efficient respiratory system; and in the last line we see that when the normally high glycolyzing system of the 3783 hepatoma competes with the 5123 hepatoma respiratory system, total phosphorylation remains very high, but over half is now respiratory phosphorylation.

These data suggest, in the light of the relative activities of pyruvate kinase in the well and poorly differentiated hepatomas, that this enzyme may well be a determinant of the glycolytic activity through competition with oxidative phosphorylation.

Competition for ADP between Pyruvate Kinase and Rat Liver Mitochondria

This conception has been documented by recent unpublished data by Mario Gosalvez (37) in our laboratory, who studied the effect of added purified pyruvate kinase on isolated, well coupled mitochondria of rat liver. A few examples of his work will illustrate the behavior of this system.

Rotenone-treated mitochondria were incubated in a vessel equipped with an oxygen electrode in the presence of varying quantities of crystalline rabbit muscle pyruvate kinase. ATP is added to serve as a source of ADP, which is continuously generated by the addition of glucose and hexokinase. As seen in the left tracing of Fig. 7, oxygen uptake markedly increased on the addition of ATP, and continued at a steady rate to exhaustion of oxygen. If, however, phosphoenolpyruvate and pyruvate kinase are added, the oxygen uptake was markedly decreased. However, when 2,4-dinitrophenol, an uncoupler of oxidative phosphorylation was added, oxygen uptake again increased. These results are interpreted

TABLE 5

Effect of Fructose-1,6-Diphosphate, (FDP) on Glycolytic and Respiratory Phosphorylation

Tissue	Substrate	2-DG Uptake	O_2 Uptake	Lactate	P resp	P glyc
Liver	None	19.7	11.5	0.9	19.7	--
	FDP	25.3	10.0	9.1	7.1	18.2
Hepatoma						
5123D	None	18.3	9.5	0	18.3	--
	FDP	23.7	10.0	3.0	17.7	6.0
3683	None	2.6	0.8	0.6	2.6	--
	FDP	28.4	3.5	13.0	2.4	26.0

TABLE 6

Effect of Intermixing Supernatants and Particles of Well and Poorly Differentiated Tumors on Glycolytic and Respiratory Phosphorylation with FDP as Substrate

Supernatant	Particles	2-DG Uptake	O_2 Uptake	Lactate	P resp	P glyc
5123	5123	18.6	9.6	1.8	15.0	3.6
3683	3683	36.0	4.2	17.6	0.8	35.2
5123	3683	27.0	4.0	13.5	~0	27.0
3683	5123	36.1	9.8	8.2	19.7	16.4

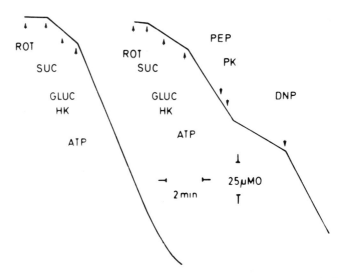

Fig. 7. *Oxygen electrode tracings illustrating inhibition of oxygen uptake by rat liver mitochondria by addition of pyruvate kinase and phosphoenolpyruvate.*

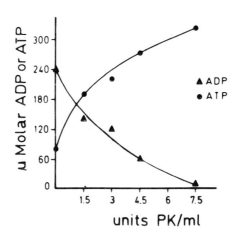

Fig. 8. *Changes in the ratio of ATP to ADP in a model system of respiring rat liver mitochondria in presence of varied amounts of pyruvate kinase.*

to indicate that pyruvate kinase can compete successfully
with the respiratory system for the available ADP, and this
interpretation has been verified in a series of similar
experiments in which the ADP levels were manipulated by
various changes in the experimental conditions.

Figure 8 demonstrates that the pyruvate kinase-induced
respiratory decrease is associated with a marked alteration
of the ratio of ATP to ADP at the steady state. In these
experiments the hexokinase concentration was 1 unit per ml
and ATP 3 mM; at these concentrations, respiratory inhibition was maximal with 7.5 units of PK per ml. A steady
state ratio was achieved after one minute as indicated by
equal ratios found after sampling at 1 min. and 4 min. of
incubation after ATP addition. The ATP/ADP ratio was about
0.3 with no PK; it was about 1 at 1 unit of PK, and increased
to 5 at 5 units of PK per ml. At the maximal O_2 inhibition
level of 7.5 units of PK per ml, the ADP level was nearly
zero. These data are thus in further accord with the view
that a major factor in determining the extents of glycolytic and respiratory phosphorylation could be the relative
activities of pyruvate kinase and the mitochondrial phosphorylation system; and that the PK activity could be a
major determinant of the ATP/ADP ratio.

On the basis of the foregoing results, we may regard
the high aerobic glycolysis of tumors, not as a *sine qua
non* of cancer, but rather as a consequence of a late stage
of dedifferentiation, possibly attributable to a molecular
form of pyruvate kinase that is at very high activity, and
is not under the same allosteric control as the isozyme of
the parent cell.

Fatty Acid Oxidation in Hepatomas

The question arises as to what the well-differentiated
tumors, which utilize glucose poorly, use for metabolic
fuel. As shown in Table 7, the answer appears to be fatty
acids. Studies from our laboratory by Bloch-Frankenthal,
et al. (38) show that oxidation of fatty acids, either to
O_2 or to acetoacetate is high in liver and in well-differentiated hepatomas, but is negligible in poorly differentiated
tumors. β-Hydroxybutyrate dehydrogenase activity, which
plays a functional role in liver in maintaining the aceto-
acetate-β-hydroxybutyrate equilibrium, and which is an important factor in the mitochondrial redox state, is moderately high in well-differentiated hepatomas, but negligible

21

TABLE 7

Fatty Acid Oxidation in Rat Hepatomas

| | Liver | Hepatomas | |
		Well differ-entiated	Poorly differ-entiated
Oxidation of Fatty Acids to CO_2	High	High	Negligible
Oxidation of Fatty Acids to Acetoacetate	High	High	Negligible
β-Hydroxybutyrate dehydrogenase Activity	High	Moderate	Negligible
Fatty Acyl CoA Synthetase Activity	High	Moderate	Low

22

in poorly-differentiated (39); and the same is true for the
first step in metabolic activation of fatty acids, their
conversion to AcylCoA (40). Thus we again see a diversity
of metabolic behavior. At the one extreme are those slow-
growing, well-differentiated hepatomas which utilize little
glucose and oxidize fatty acids; and at the other extreme
are those rapidly growing, poorly differentiated hepatomas,
that have largely lost the capability for fatty acid oxidation, but have acquired the ability to utilize glucose.

Discussion

The Morris hepatomas have taught us that a single
cell type of origin can give rise to tumors of great diversity, paralleled by diversity in the molecular structures
of their enzymes. It is now clear that mere assays of total
enzyme activity do not reveal profound alterations in isozyme activity which undoubtedly affect the metabolism and
growth of these hepatomas. It may be considered as a
general proposition that the loss of those isozymes that
are under host regulation and that are geared to organ function, and their replacement by isozymes geared to the efficient utilization of metabolic fuels represent the molecular
basis for the unbridled proliferation of tumors.
Obviously, these studies of a few enzymes of carbohydrate and fatty acid metabolism only scratch the surface
of what is in all likelihood a general phenomenon of neoplasia. Experiments of others indicate that similar izo-
zyme alterations in hepatomas, with expression of fetal
isozymes, occur with various aminotransferases (41), glutaminase (42), thymidine kinase (43), and probably other
enzymes.

Alterations in Antigens

There is a striking similarity between these isozyme
alterations and the alterations in immunologic properties.
In cancer, antigens specific to the adult differentiated
cells disappear, while new tumor-associated antigens appear;
in many instances these neoantigens are present also in
fetal tissue. The elaboration of a fetal protein, the so-
called carcinoembryonic antigen, in tumors of the gastrointestinal tract (8,44) offers the exciting promise of early
clinical diagnosis. The so called gs (group specific)

antigen found in many mouse tumors induced by oncogenic C-type viruses, is also present in fetal tissues (45). According to the oncogene hypothesis, the viral genome is integrated with the host DNA and is thus genetically transmitted. The presence of this antigen in tumors is another instance of the activation in tumors of a fetal protein. Rapp and others (46) have shown in SV-40 viral transformed hamster cells a surface antigen is derived from the host cell genome which is also found in hamster embryos; and Baldwin (47) has observed fetal antigens in chemically-induced rat hepatomas.

In considering the underlying cause of the expression of embryonic proteins in tumors, another question arises as to whether this is programmed or fortuitous. These embryonic manifestations have been described in such terms as derepressive dedifferentiation (8), retrogenic expression (8, 44,11), retrodifferentiation (7), blocked ontogeny (48), etc., implying a more or less systematic reversion to an embryonic state; that is, a reversal of normal ontogeny. Our isozyme data do indicate some order in the observed alterations. For example, many well-differentiated hepatomas have largely lost isozymes of the differentiated liver cell but do not exhibit a resurgence of the fetal isozyme; but when resurgence of the fetal form does occur, there is always a loss of the normal hepatic isozyme (18). These observations suggest that certain genes may have to be switched off before others are switched on. However, in general the alterations seem to be sporadic and unpredictable, and therefore suggest a disordered rather than a programmed mechanism of gene activation.

Ectopic Protein Synthesis

This conception of a disordered rather than a programmed reversion is strongly bolstered by a large and ever-growing body of clinical literature pointing to bizarre aberrations of protein synthesis in certain tumors, resulting in the ectopic production of polypeptide hormones (1-4).

Such profound anomalies of gene expression are striking in view of the normally highly selective control of gene transcription in normal differentiated tissue and raise many questions concerning their significance to neoplasia. It is attractive to consider that neoplasia is initiated by some impairment of this regulatory mechanism. Once the rigid control is lost, many of the familiar patterns of neoplasia would inevitably follow; chromosome aber-

24

rations, loss of antigens, alterations in surface properties, and all of the other characteristics of tumor progression could be envisioned to result from this initial injury. Considerable discussion surrounds the question whether cancer is due to a somatic mutation. The present work, especially in light of the alterations in antigens, points to a disorder of gene expression rather than of gene structure. Arguing also against somatic mutation is the fact that the abnormal proteins which arise in tumors are not "new" protein species, but rather are "misplaced" proteins; misplaced either in site, as exemplified by the ectopic production of polypeptide hormones; or in time, as exemplified by the resurgence of fetal proteins in the form of isozymes and antigens. If cancer results from a somatic mutation it would appear to be a mutation of a regulatory rather than a structural gene.

The field of cancer research is a graveyard of abortive theories and hypotheses; and it is important to ask whether these aberrations of protein synthesis are the cause or the effect of the neoplastic transformation. Neither isozyme nor antigen alterations are all or none phenomena; but rather are quantitative; many of the isozymes normally vary greatly, depending on dietary or hormonal conditions; some antigens at least appear in regenerating and aging tissue as well as in fetal liver; and many of the isozyme alterations seen in poorly differentiated hepatomas also appear in ostensibly normal liver cells grown *in vitro* (49). Many more questions can be asked and one can speculate at great length in the light of these anomalies of gene expression; obviously we need more information on the mechanisms of normal differentiation before we can understand these disorders of differentiation, which may lie at the heart of the neoplastic transformation.

Summary

Studies of enzyme activities and isoenzyme composition in the Morris hepatomas, a series of chemically induced, transplantable rat hepatomas ranging widely in growth rate and degree of differentiation, have revealed a common pattern of isozyme alteration. In the highly differentiated, slow growing hepatomas the sole or preponderant isozymes are the so-called liver marker types; *e.g.*, glucokinase, aldolase B, pyruvate kinase L, and the liver-type glycogen

25

phosphorylase. With decreased differentiation and increased
growth rate, these liver types decrease markedly; and in
the fast growing, poorly differentiated hepatomas, the liver
type isozymes are nearly or completely replaced by high
activities of non-hepatic type isozymes. The slow growing,
well-differentiated hepatomas utilize glucose poorly and
have a low rate of aerobic glycolysis; but like normal adult
liver they utilize fatty acids as respiratory fuel. The
fast growing, poorly differentiated hepatomas have largely
lost the ability to oxidize fatty acids, but have a high
aerobic glycolysis and utilize glucose as a respiratory
fuel.

Evidence from experiments in model systems points to
the high levels of pyruvate kinase as a determining factor
in the high aerobic glycolysis in the poorly differentiated
hepatomas. It is proposed that the replacement of isozymes
geared for organ function by isozymes, geared primarily for
efficient utilization of metabolites and that are not under
host dietary or endocrine control, represents a molecular
basis for the uncontrolled proliferation of cancer cells.

These findings are similar to other aberrancies of
protein synthesis in cancer, such as the loss of tissue-
specific antigens and the appearance of tumor-associated
antigens, and the "ectopic" production of polypeptide hormones by non-endocrine neoplasms. The isozyme data thus
support and add functional significance to an ever-increas-
ing body of evidence for an anomaly of gene expression in
cancer, whereby certain genes that code for proteins present in normal adult tissue are switched off and genes
that are normally inactive are switched on. The fact that
antigens and isozymes found in tumors are also present in
fetal tissues suggests that genes active in the fetal stage
but inactivated during normal embryonic development are
re-activated in cancer.

*Presented by Sidney Weinhouse. The experimental work
of the authors is currently being supported by grants CA-
12227 and CA-10916 from the National Cancer Institute and
BC-74 from the American Cancer Society. The collaboration
of Dr. Harold P. Morris in this work is gratefully acknow-
ledged, as is also the association in this work of Dr.
Kiyomi Sato, Jennie Shatton and Mario Gosalvez. The author
wishes to thank Cancer Research for permission to use Fig.
4 and Science for Fig. 2.*

References

1. Eliel, L.P. Non-endocrine secreting neoplasms: Clinical manifestations. Cancer Bull. 20: 37-39 (1968).
2. Goodall, C.M. A review: On para-endocrine cancer syndromes. Int'l. J. of Cancer 4: 1-10 (1969).
3. Lipsett, M.B. Humoral syndromes associated with non-endocrine tumors. Ann. Int'l Med. 61: 733-756 (1964).
4. Roof, B.S., B. Carpenter, D.J. Fink and G.S. Gordon. Some thoughts on the nature of ectopic parathyroid hormones. Am. J. Med. 50: 686-691 (1971).
5. Abelev, G.I. α-Fetoprotein in oncogenesis and its association with malignant tumors. Advances in Cancer Res. 14: 195-358 (1971).
6. Alexander, P. Foetal "antigens" in cancer. Nature 235: 137-140 (1972).
7. Anderson, N.G. and J.H. Coggin, Jr. Models of differentiation, retrogression and cancer. Proceedings of the First Conference on Embryonic and Fetal Antigens in Cancer. Oak Ridge National Laboratory (1971), pp. 7-37.
8. Gold, P. Embryonic origin of human tumor-specific antigens. Prog. Exp. Tumor. Res. 14: 43-58 (1971).
9. Lengerova, L. Expression of normal histocompatability antigens in tumor cells. Adv. Cancer Res. 16: 235-272 (1972).
10. Stanislawski-Birencwajg, M., J. Uriel and P. Grabar. Association of embryonic antigens with experimentally induced hepatic lesions in the rat. Cancer Res. 27: 1990-1997 (1967).
11. Stonehill, E.H. and A. Bendich. The reappearance of embryonal antigens in cancer cells. Nature 228: 370-371 (1970).
12. Uriel, J. Transitory liver antigens and primary hepatoma in man and rat. Path. Biol. 17: 877: 884 (1969).
13. Criss, W.E. A review of isozymes in cancer. Cancer Res. 31: 1523-1542 (1971).
14. Knox, W.E. Enzyme patterns in fetal, adult and neoplastic rat tissues. S. Karger AG., Basel (1972).
15. Ono, T. and S. Weinhouse (Editors). Isozymes and Enzyme Regulation in Cancer. Gann Monograph, Vol. 13, Univ. of Tokyo Press (1972).
16. Shapira, F., M.D. Reuber and A. Hatzfeld. Resurgence of two fetal-type aldolases (A and C) in some fast-growing hepatomas. Biochem. Biophys. Res. Commun. 40:

321-325 (1970).

17. Schapira, F. Isozymes in cancer. Advances in Cancer Res. 18 (in press).

18. Weinhouse, S. Glycolysis, respiration and anomalous gene expression in experimental hepatomas: G.H.A. Clowes Memorial Lecture. Cancer Res. 32: 2007-2016 (1972).

19. Morris, H.P. Some growth morphological and biochemical characteristics of hepatoma 5123 and other transplantable hepatomas. Prog. Exp. Tumor Res. 3: 370-411 (1963).

20. Morris, H.P. Studies on the development, biochemistry and biology of experimental hepatomas. Advances in Cancer Res. 9: 227-302 (1965).

21. Morris, H.P. and B.P. Wagner. Induction and transplantation of rat hepatomas with different growth rate (including minimal deviation hepatomas). In: H. Busch (Editor), Methods in Cancer Res. Academic Press, New York (1968), Vol. 4, pp. 125-152.

22. Aisenberg, A.C. and H.P. Morris. Energy pathways of hepatomas 5123. Nature, 191: 1314-1316 (1961).

23. Elwood, J.C., Y.C. Lin, V.J. Cristofalo, S. Weinhouse and H.P. Morris. Glucose utilization in homogenates of the Morris Hepatoma 5123 and related tumors. Cancer Res. 23: 906-913 (1963).

24. Weber, G., G. Banerjee and H.P. Morris. Comparative biochemistry of hepatomas. I. Carbohydrate enzymes in Morris Hepatoma 5123. Cancer Res. 21: 933-937 (1961).

25. Sato, K., H.P. Morris and S. Weinhouse. Phosphorylase: A new isozyme in rat hepatic tumors and fetal liver. Science 178: 879-881 (1972).

26. Sato, K., H.P. Morris and S. Weinhouse. Characterization of glycogen synthetases and phosphorylases in transplantable rat hepatomas. Cancer Res. 33: 724-733 (1973).

27. Sato, K. and S. Weinhouse. Purification and characterization of the Novikoff Hepatoma glycogen phosphorylase and its relations to a fetal form. Arch. Biochem. Biophys. (in press) (1973).

28. Farina, F., J.B. Shatton, H.P. Morris and S. Weinhouse. Unpublished work.

29. Warburg, O. The Metabolism of Tumors. Arnold Constable, London (1930).

30. Weinhouse, S. Studies on the fate of isotopically labeled metabolites in the oxidative metabolism of tumors. Cancer Res. 11: 585-591 (1951).
31. Aisenberg, A.C. The Glycolysis and Respiration of Tumors. Academic Press, New York (1961).
32. Newsholme, A.E. and W. Gevers. Control of glycolysis and gluconeogenesis in liver and kidney cortex. Vitamins and Hormones 25: 1-79 (1967).
33. Passoneau, J.V. and O.H. Lowry. The role of phospho-fructokinase in metabolic regulation. Advan. Enzyme Regulation 2: 265-276 (1964).
34. Johnson, M.J. The role of aerobic phosphorylation in the Pasteur Effect. Science 94: 200-202 (1941).
35. Lynen, F. The aerobic phosphate requirement of yeast. The Pasteur Effect. Ann. Chem. 546: 120-141 (1941).
36. Lo, C.H., V.J. Cristofalo, H.P. Morris and S. Weinhouse. Studies on respiration and glycolysis in transplanted hepatomas of the rat. Cancer Res. 18: 1-10 (1968).
37. Gosalvez, M., J. Perez-Garcia and S. Weinhouse. Unpublished work.
38. Bloch-Frankenthal, L., J. Langan, H.P. Morris and S. Weinhouse. Fatty acid oxidation and ketogenesis in transplantable liver tumors. Cancer Res. 25: 732-736 (1965).
39. Ohe, K., H.P. Morris and S. Weinhouse. β-Hydroxy-butyrate dehydrogenase activity in liver and liver tumors. Cancer Res. 27: 1360-1371 (1967).
40. Langan, J., H.P. Morris and S. Weinhouse. Unpublished work.
41. Ichihara, A. and K. Ogawa. Isozymes of branched chain amino acid transaminase in normal rat tissues and hepatomas. Gann Monograph. 13: 181-190 (1972).
42. Katunuma, N., T. Katsunuma, I. Tomino and Y. Matsuda. Regulation of glutaminase activity and differentiation of the isozyme during development. Advan. Enzyme Regulation 6: 227-242 (1968).
43. Jones, O.W., A. Taylor and M.A. Stafford. Fetal gene expression in human tumor cells. J. Clin. Invest. 51: 47a (1972).
44. Gold, P. and S.O. Freedman. Specific carcinoembryonic antigens of the human digestive tract. J. Exp. Med. 122: 467-481 (1965).
45. Huebner, R.J., G.J. Kelloff, P.S. Sarma, W.T. Lane, H.C. Turner, R.V. Gilden, S. Oroszlan, H. Meyer, D.D. Myers and R.L. Peters. Group-specific antigen expres-

SIDNEY WEINHOUSE

RNA tumor virus: Implications for ontogenesis and
oncogenesis. Proc. Nat. Acad. Sci. USA 67: 336–376
(1970).

46. Duff, R. and F. Rapp. Reaction of serum from pregnant
hamsters with surface of cells transormed by SV-40
J. Immunol. 105: 521–523 (1970).

47. Baldwin, R.W. Immunological aspects of chemical
carcinogenesis. Advances in Cancer Res. (in press)
(1973).

48. Potter, V.R. Environmentally-induced metabolic oscil-
lations as a challenge to tumor autonomy. Miami
Winter Symposium, North Holland, Amsterdam, 2: 291–
313 (1970).

49. Farber, E., J.B. Shatton and S. Weinhouse. Unpublished
work.

30

REGULATION OF GENE EXPRESSION AND VIRAL NEOPLASIA

Francis T. Kenney, Kai-Lin Lee and James N. Ihle

Introduction

Hormonal regulation of synthesis of tyrosine aminotransferase and activation of production of leukemia viruses would
appear to have little in common. But from the vantage point
of gene regulation they may be quite comparable, for both
appear to be instances where nature has provided for close
regulation of the expression of specific components of the
genome of the mammalian cell. The tyrosine aminotransferase
system has served as a convenient model to probe mechanisms
controlling transcription (induction by glucocorticoids),
translation (insulin induction), and other aspects of regulation in mammalian cells; information derived from the
analysis of this and other examples of hormonally regulated
gene expression is beginning to provide a firm foundation
for a full understanding of mammalian genetic regulation.
However, mammalian genetic regulation is of more than academic interest. Evidence is accumulating (1,2) that some
and perhaps all cancers may be specified by genes associated
with RNA tumor virus genomes inherited as part of the natural
DNA component of the cells. This view suggests that defects
or breakdowns in regulation of selected genes is associated
with the onset of cancers, *i.e.*, cancer is a disease of gene
expression, and the significant genes may be associated with
expression of RNA tumor viruses. In this paper we will
summarize some of our recent results on transcriptional regulation of the model aminotransferase system as well as those
from preliminary approaches to the regulation of virus
expression.

Results and Discussion

Transcriptional Control of Tyrosine Aminotransferase

31

In recent papers we have presented data and summarized evidence in support of the view that glucocorticoids induce tyrosine aminotransferase by specifically accelerating synthesis of enzyme-specific mRNA (3-5). Briefly, this can be recapitulated as follows (*see,* Fig. 1): (1) degradative rate λ_1 and λ_2 of the enzyme and its mRNA are unchanged by hydrocortisone treatment; (2) the rate of enzyme synthesis is specifically increased; (3) the kinetics of induction by hydrocortisone are those expected if Nt, the cellular content of enzyme specific mRNA, is increased by the hormone; (4) induction is prevented by inhibitors of RNA synthesis. To these points we might add the evidence that induction requires a nuclear-localizing complex of hormone with a receptor protein (6,7) and that induction is prevented by concentrations of cordecypin which specifically inhibit maturation (adenylation) of mRNA (8).

We specifically reject the argument that inducing steroids act post-transcriptionally to antagonize a repressor that inhibits translation and promotes mRNA degradation (9). The rate of mRNA degradation is not changed by steroid inducers (4). Further, this argument is based on the contention that, when cells are pretreated with steroid and then with high concentrations of actinomycin, the "paradoxical" increase (or maintenance of) the enzyme level that occurs is due to increased (or maintained) rates of enzyme synthesis. Our analyses have consistently shown that enzyme synthesis is inhibited under these conditions; the enzyme level is increased (or maintained) by virtue of an actinomycin-mediated block of enzyme degradation (4,8).

It will be noted that none of the points made above constitute direct proof for our contention that steroids act to regulate transcriptional events. This requires isolation and quantitation of each of the macromolecules depicted in Fig. 1. We have initiated attempts to isolate the aminotransferase-specific mRNA, using a combination of the immunological techniques introduced by Schimke *et al.* (10), and a newly developed chromatography method wherein mRNAs can be fractionated by virtue of differences in their polyadenylate content (11).

In Fig. 2 are presented preliminary results of experiments wherein aminotransferase-specific polysomes were precipitated from total hepatoma cell polysomes with anti-aminotransferase serum. The RNA species of the precipitable fraction (<2% of the total) and of the fraction not precipitated were obtained by phenol extraction and subjected to

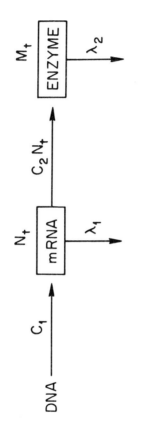

Fig. 1. *Model of cellular events controlling enzyme levels in mammalian cells.*

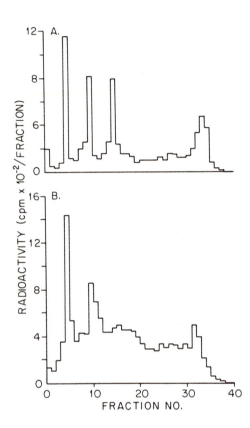

Fig. 2. *Gel electrophoretic analysis of RNA species of polysome fractions.* Hydrocortisone-treated H-35 cells were labeled with ^{32}P (1 mCi/ml) for 2 hr., then collected and lysed with 0.5% Triton. Polysomes were prepared by the method of Blobel and Potter (18), and RNA extracted with phenol at pH 9. (A) RNA from the fraction of polysomes precipitated by the F(ab')$_2$ fragment of antiaminotransferase antibody. (B) RNA from the fraction (>98%) not precipitated with antibody.

electrophoresis on acrylamide gels. The fraction not precipitated resembles the total preparation and contains distinct 28, 18 and 4–5S species as well as a great deal of
RNA with S values ranging from 5 to 20S. In contrast, the
precipitated polysomes contain primarily one RNA species in
addition to ribosomal and transfer RNAs (*i.e.*, 28, 18 and
4–5S RNAs). This species is 14–15S, which is the size expected for the mRNA coding for the aminotransferase subunit
(assuming four subunits, each of about 220 amino acids) and
containing in addition about 100 adenylate residues.

 This RNA can be further purified by hybridization to,
and controlled elution from, columns of poly (U)-Sepharose.
Stepwise increments in elution temperature, after hybridization is complete, successfully fractionates adenylate poly-
mers containing 15 to 200 residues; chain length is essentially linear with increasing temperature between these
limits (11). Fractionation of total polysomal mRNA from
hepatoma cells, using this technique, is shown in Fig. 3.
It is apparent that the polyadenylate content of this mRNA
is not constant, but ranges from 20 to 30 residues (22°) to
150 residues (40°), with the bulk of the RNAs containing
100 to 150 adenylate residues.

 These procedures hold the promise that isolation of
specific mRNAs from mammalian cells, even those coding for
minor cellular proteins like tyrosine aminotransferase, will
soon be routine. We are in the process of scaling our isolation procedures up to the level required to prepare the
apparently specific mRNA species in quantity sufficient to
determine if it does, indeed, code specifically for tyrosine
aminotransferase. Once this is established the question of
transcriptional *vs* translational control in the hormonal
regulation of this enzyme should be readily answered.

 Figure 3 also demonstrates the fractionation on poly(U)-
Sepharose of the RNA genome of murine leukemia virus (12).
Green and Cartas (13) and Ross *et al.* (14) have shown that
the intact 70S RNA genome of murine oncogenic RNA viruses,
like the mRNAs of mammalian cells, contain poly(A). The
70S RNA is disrupted by mild heating, yielding 3 to 4 36S
subunits and a small amount of low molecular weight RNA.
Fractionation of the 36S subunits on poly(U)-Sepharose re-
veals that roughly half elute at 20° (*i.e.*, fail to hybridize
under these conditions) and thus contain no poly(A) regions
of more than 15–20 residues. The remainder elutes as a
homogeneous peak at 44–46°, corresponding to RNA having
poly(A) regions of approximately 175 adenylate residues.

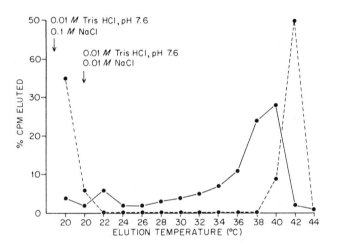

Fig. 3. *Fractionation of polysomal and leukemia virus RNA on polyuridylate-Sepharose columns.* Polysomal RNA from H-35 cells (solid line), prepared as in the legend to Fig. 2, and the 36S subunits of Moloney leukemia virus RNA (broken line), prepared as described in the text, were hybridized to columns of poly(U)-Sepharose and then eluted with increasing temperature.

This result suggests that the poly(A)-containing and nonpoly (A)-containing fractions represent genetically distinct components of the viral genome, a question which is now being studied.

Regulation of Virus Expression

Perhaps the most impressive experimental support for the view that the information for RNA tumor viruses is normally present in cells in "repressed" form, is the demonstration by Rowe et al. (15) that cultured virus-free cells can be made to begin producing virus by treatment with agents such as halogenated pyrimidines. We have begun a study of the physiological requirements for virus expression in the AKR cell system of Rowe et al., as a beginning approach to the molecular mechanisms involved.

Table 1 shows the results of experiments in which we asked whether iododeoxyuridine (IdUrd) treatment of AKR cells results in the formation of an intermediate of some stability. These cells cease DNA synthesis and cell replication shortly after serum is withdrawn from the medium. If serum is not provided over the four day course of the experiment following 24 hr. exposure to IdUrd, no activation is observed, confirming the demonstration by Rowe et al. (15) that synthesis of DNA is required. However these data also show that serum can be withheld for 1, 2, or 3 days after IdUrd treatment; when DNA synthesis is restored by serum addition at these times, virus expression is observed. Thus IdUrd treatment results in the formation of a stable intermediate which requires synthesis of DNA before full expression of the virus can occur.

These results are reminiscent of those reported by Temin (16), who found that exogenous infection with avian sarcoma viruses results in the formation of a DNA "provirus"; full expression of the "provirus" requires DNA synthesis and cell replication. Comparable results can be seen with exogenous murine tumor virus infection of 3T3 cells (Fig. 4). If DNA synthesis is prevented by removal of serum after the cells are infected no virus is synthesized, but virus expression can be recovered up to 4 days later by restoration of capacity to synthesize DNA.

The implication of a two stage mechanism in the activation of virus expression in AKR cells by IdUrd was further examined with specific inhibitors. Here thymidine (at low concentration) was used as a competitor with IdUrd for in-

37

TABLE 1

Stability of Iododeoxyuridine-Effected Change
in AKR Cells During Virus Activation

Treatment[a]	% Cells Positive
Serum present throughout	4.84
No serum after IdUrd; 1, 2, 3, or 4 days	0.00
Serum immediately after IdUrd	3.72
Serum 1 day after IdUrd	3.14
Serum 2 days after IdUrd	4.13
Serum 3 days after IdUrd	2.17

[a]AKR cells were treated with IdUrd (100 µg/ml) for 24 hr.
under conditions permitting DNA synthesis. After this exposure synthesis of DNA was blocked by removal of serum or
restored by serum addition immediately or 1, 2, or 3 days
later. The fraction of cells synthesizing leukemia virus
was determined by fluorescent antibody techniques 48 hr.
after serum addition or withdrawl.

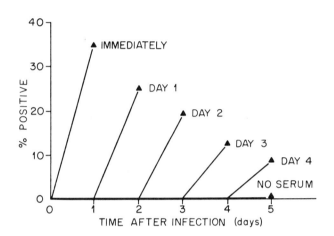

Fig. 4. *Stability of "provirus" formed after infection of 3T3 cells with Moloney leukemia virus.* Cells were deprived of serum 12 hr. prior to infection on day 0. Serum was added immediately or 1, 2, 3 or 4 days after virus, and the fraction of cells synthesizing virus determined by fluorescent antibody techniques 24 hr. later.

corporation into DNA, colchicine as a mitotic block, and
cytosine arabinoside as an inhibitor of DNA synthesis. In
these experiments the cells were deprived of serum for a
short time before and during IdUrd treatment; under these
conditions DNA synthesis is possible during the period of
treatment but stops soon thereafter. After IdUrd treatment
was completed, serum was restored to permit recovery of
synthesis of DNA. The results (Table 2) show that cytosine
arabinoside, if added either during or after IdUrd treatment, completely blocks virus expression; thus, DNA synthesis is required for both stages. Thymidine inhibits only
if added during the period of IdUrd treatment, in confirma-
tion of the observations of Teich *et al.* (17) suggesting
that IdUrd must be incorporated into DNA to activate virus
expression. Colchicine blocks expression if added at either
time, suggesting that chromosome replication as well as
synthesis of DNA is required for each stage.

We interpret these data as indicating that activation
of endogenous leukemia virus is a two stage process. In the
initial stage IdUrd is incorporated into cellular DNA,
perhaps causing its breakdown or otherwise "derepressing"
the viral genes. After incorporation of IdUrd a stable
intermediate is formed which may be comparable or identical
to the "provirus" formed when cells are infected by exogenous virus. Expression of the intermediate as production
of extracellular virus requires another round of DNA synthesis and chromosome replication. These relationships are
depicted graphically in Fig. 5, which we propose as a working model from which further understanding of the mechanisms
involved in virus expression may be gained.

---

*Presented by Francis T. Kenney, Carcinogenesis Program,
Biology Division, Oak Ridge National Laboratory, Oak Ridge,
Tennessee, 37830. Research supported jointly by the Virus
Cancer Program of the National Cancer Institute and by the
U.S. Atomic Energy Commission under contract with Union
Carbide Corporation.*

References

1. Huebner, R.J. and G.J. Todaro. Oncogenes of RNA tumor
    viruses as determinants of cancer. Proc. Nat. Acad. Sci.
    USA 64: 1087-1094 (1969).

TABLE 2

Effects of Inhibitors on Leukemia Virus Expression
in Iododeoxyuridine-Treated AKR Cells

Inhibitor Added[a]	% Cells Positive
None	2.38
Cytosine arabinoside with IdUrd	0.00
Cytosine arabinoside with serum	0.00
Colchicine with IdUrd	0.00
Colchicine with serum	0.00
Thymidine with IdUrd	0.00
Thymidine with serum	2.14

[a]AKR cells were deprived of serum 6 hr. prior to and during treatment with IdUrd (100 μg, 24 hr.; first stage). Serum was restored after removal of IdUrd, and after 48 hr. (second stage) the fraction of cells synthesizing leukemia virus was determined using fluorescent antibody techniques. Inhibitors were added in first or second stages as indicated. Concentrations: cytosine arabinoside, 0.5 mM; colchicine, 1 μM; thymidine, 24 μg/ml.

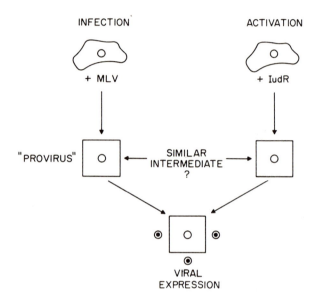

INFECTION
ACTIVATION

+ MLV
+ IudR

"PROVIRUS"
SIMILAR
INTERMEDIATE
?

VIRAL
EXPRESSION

Fig. 5. *Suggested relationship between exogenous viral infection and activation of endogenous virus.*

2. Todaro, G.J. and R.J. Huebner. The viral oncogene
hypothesis: New evidence. Proc. Nat. Acad. Sci. USA
69: 1009-1015 (1972).
3. Reel, J.R., K.-L. Lee and F.T. Kenney. Regulation of
tyrosine-α-ketoglutarate transaminase in rat liver.
VIII. Inductions by hydrocortisone and insulin in
cultured hepatoma cells. J. Biol. Chem. 245: 5800-
5805 (1970).
4. Lee, K.-L., J.R. Reel and F.T. Kenney. Regulation of
tyrosine-α-ketoglutarate transaminase in rat liver.
IX. Studies of the mechanisms of hormonal inductions
in cultured hepatoma cells. J. Biol. Chem. 245: 5806-
5812 (1970).
5. Kenney, F.T., K.-L. Lee and K.L. Barker. Hormonal
mechanisms in regulation of gene expression. In:
Gene Expression and Its Regulation, F.T. Kenney, B.A.
Hamkalo, G. Favelukes and J.T. August, (Editors).
Plenum Press, New York, pp. 487-502.
6. Baxter, J.D. and G.M. Tomkins. The relationship between glucocorticoid binding and tyrosine aminotransferase induction in hepatoma tissue culture cells.
Proc. Nat. Acad. Sci. USA 65: 709-714 (1970).
7. Kenney, F.T. and K.-L. Lee. Regulation of enzyme synthesis in cultured cells by adrenal steroids. Excerpta
Med. Internat. Cong. Series 219: 472-478 (1970).
8. Lee, K.-L., C.D. Stiles, J.E. Fritz and F.T. Kenney.
Manuscript in preparation.
9. Tomkins, G.M., T.D. Gelehrter, D.K. Granner, D.M.
Martin Jr., H.H. Samuels and E.G. Thompson. Control
of specific gene expression in higher organisms.
Science 166: 1474-1479 (1969).
10. Schimke, R.T., R. Palacios, R.D. Palmiter and R.E.
Thoads. Hormonal regulation of ovalbumin synthesis in
chick oviduct. In: Gene Expression and Its Regulation,
F.T. Kenney, B.A. Hamkalo, G. Favelukes and J.T. August,
(Editors). Plenum Press, New York, pp. 123-136.
11. Lee, K.-L. and D.R. Joseph. Manuscript in preparation.
12. Ihle, J.N., K.-L. Lee and F.T. Kenney. Manuscript in
preparation.
13. Green, M. and M. Cartas. The genome of RNA tumor viruses contains polyadenylic acid sequences. Proc. Nat.
Acad. Sci. USA 69: 791-794 (1972).
14. Ross, J., S.R. Tronick and E.M. Scolnick. Polyadeny-
late-rich RNA in the 70S RNA of murine leukemia-sarcoma
virus. Virol. 49: 230-235 (1972).

15. Rowe, W.P., D.R. Lowry, N. Teich and J.W. Hartley. Some implications of the activation of murine leukemia virus by halogenated pyrimidines. Proc. Nat. Acad. Sci. USA 69: 1033-1035 (1972).
16. Temin, H.M. Studies on carcinogenesis by avian sarcoma viruses. V. Requirement for new DNA synthesis and cell division. J. Cell. Physiol. 69: 53-64 (1967).
17. Teich, N., D.R. Lowry, J.W. Hartley and W.P. Rowe. Studies of the mechanism of induction of infectious murine leukemia virus from AKR mouse embryo cell lines by 5-iododeoxyuridine and 5-bromodeoxyuridine. Virol. 51: 163-173 (1973).
18. Blobel, G. and V.R. Potter. Ribosomes in rat liver: an estimate of the percentage of free and membrane-bound ribosomes interacting with messenger RNA *in vivo*. J. Mol. Biol. 28: 539-542 (1969).

THE CHEMICAL PROTOTYPE OF TUMORS IN RELATION TO THE COMPO-
SITIONS OF RAT TISSUES

W. Eugene Knox

Introduction

Investigations have recently begun to demonstrate some
order among neoplasms, at least among those experimental
tumors of the rat that are most often studied by biochemists.
Before this, biochemistry contributed to cancer research a
succession of fragile hypotheses -- D-glutamate in tumor
proteins, defective tumor respiration, or unique constituents of tumors, which after enormous effort were one by
one proved to be illusory. Failures rather than knowledge
accumulated. In consequence, neoplasms are still considered
by many to be chemically bizarre and disordered growths,
even in the face of evidence that they do grow and reproduce
only too efficiently. Biochemical "successes" in cancer
research will remain essentially negative in character
until the orderliness, and not the disorder, of tumors is
studied.

A modest beginning is the evidence to be presented here
that a limited spectrum of tumors share a common composition,
akin to that of normal fetal tissues. The quantitative
chemical similarities between tumors and immature tissues
fit their functional likenesses. The qualitative similarity
of many specific isozymes in tumors and immature tissues
also shows that there is reactivation in tumors of a significant portion of the cell's fetal genome. Constructive hypotheses instead of only null hypotheses about the nature of
neoplasms can now be tested.

Histological Characterization of Neoplasia

Morphological identification and classification is the
rock upon which our knowledge of neoplasia rests, inadequate
though that may seem to some. Constructive chemical ideas
about the nature of neoplasms can reasonably be expected to

45

accord with what is already known of the morphological
characteristics of tumors. Chemical information that cannot be related to the morphological experience of a hundred
years may indeed by irrelevant to the nature of neoplasia.
Initially, at least, chemical information must be used in
a special way to meet this elementary criterion of relevance
to the only coherent knowledge of tumors we now have.

Morphology teaches us that neoplasms are altered cells
of the host -- flesh of our flesh -- which can (usually) be
classified as coming from one or another of the normal
tissues of the body. Those coming from any single tissue
are found to grade from nearly normal, well-differentiated
tumors up to such undifferentiated tumors that classification as to origin is not possible. In general, "malignancy"
or neoplasticity increases with the higher grades of tumor
dedifferentiation and faster rates of growth. The spectrum
of graded tumors from any one tissue type and the many types
of normal tissues that can become neoplastic produces a
very great variety of neoplasms. Each tumor may in fact
be unique, and if so, the efficiency of the histological
classification system is all the more impressive for containing in a practical way an almost infinite variety of
tumors.

Can biochemical, as opposed to histological characterization, confirm or even extend this successful scheme for
recognizing and classifying tumors? Quantitative chemical
analysis is a powerful tool of very high resolution. It
can demonstrate numerical relations or differences between
tissues. The kinds of analyses used can be multiplied to
whatever extent is necessary to reveal even minor distinctions. It is necessary only to express the different components on the same scale so that they can be compared. The
averaged chemical differences of a number of components
measured in any two tissues can be expressed as a number,
and this can be graphed as the "chemical distance" between
the tissues. A map is produced of the relationships among
tissues. If the histological characteristics upon which
microscopists rely could be quantified, the "histological
distances" between tissues and tumors could also be graphed
in an exactly analogous manner. This would show the structure of the classification system already described. In
fact, no such numbers exist, but a diagram of the classification will show its principle, and also show that it has
unresolved ambiguities. Pathologists divide fairly equally
between favoring one or another of the two possible concep-

tual structures shown in Fig. 1. The difference between the structures is not trivial. It would be important for biochemistry merely to confirm the general nature of these conceptual structures derived from histology. It would be a significant scientific advance to identify which one is correct.

I have assumed in these conceptual structures that there is a graded relationship between different tumors of a single tissue type, because such gradations are supported by strong histological and clinical evidence for a number of important kinds of human tumors, and because chemical grading of the rat hepatomas has been a major result of recent biochemical endeavor. Gradation within a single tumor type is shown diagrammatically in the figure by the linear, monotonic departure of tumors (open circles) farther and farther from their tissue of origin (solid circle). The differences ("distances") between tumor and parent tissue become greater for the higher grade tumors. Both conceptual structures also show distances among the several tissues of origin, reflecting the familiar differences, histological and chemical, that exist among liver, kidney, skin and so on.

The crucial difference between the two conceptual structures in Fig. 1 is that the tissue-tumor relations in the "unique" structure are peculiar for each tissue (shown by the tumors lying in different directions from their tissues of origin). In the second "concerted" structure all tumors depart in the same general direction from the several normal tissues. If the first structure were correct, neoplasia of each tissue would constitute an individual problem, with its own nature and means of diagnosis and treatment, and little transfer of information between problems could occur. The second structure offers a more general set of solutions that would be applicable to tumors of many kinds of tissues. The success of a pathologist in recognizing many kinds of tumors, including ones from tissues not previously seen by him, suggests that some general solutions do exist.

It is important to note a variant of the second conceptual structure (indicated by dashed lines). Here tumors depart in nearly the same direction from the normal tissues, but in such a way that the higher grade tumors actually become more like one another. This subsidiary scheme could explain why even the most experienced pathologists sometimes cannot identify the cellular origin of a particular tumor.

47

The highest grade tumors (labelled "prototypic") will have lost most of the characteristics of normal tissues and thereby simply will have become indistinguishable. Such chemical similarity between tumors from different sources (all probably of high grade) was in fact demonstrated by J.P. Greenstein a quarter of a century ago (1; Summary and references in 2, Chaps. I and II). Fig. 2 shows Greenstein's summary (3) of the chemical similarities among different mouse tumors and the contrasting chemical diversities found among normal tissues. This uniformity of the chemical compositions of different kinds of tumors contradicted the general appreciation that there was extreme biological diversity to be found among neoplasms. One solution to this still unresolved paradox of uniformity *versus* diversity among tumors is inherent in the subsidiary second diagram of Fig. 1. Uniformity exists among the high grade tumors. Diversity exists among the lower grade tumors. There is dissimilarity between two tumors that are each closely related to a different normal tissue, and also among those tumors of different grades from a single tissue.

This brief review of the one coherent body of information about the nature of neoplasms, that of morphology, shows that important alternatives in its conceptual scheme remain. Biochemical information is compatible with that of morphology in the single, well-investigated case of the different grades of hepatomas. During the past decade the orderly chemical gradation found among tumors of this single organ has been firmly established under the leadership of Weber (4,5). Any single line in any version of the schemes in Fig. 1 can represent this relationship among liver and the hepatomas. For this single tissue-tumor system biochemistry is in accord with histology. This is an important achievement for biochemistry, even if it is not an advance for oncology.

The chemical uniformity among different kinds of tumors as reported by Greenstein remains paradoxical, but it could be fitted into one of the alternatives still open in the morphological scheme. Specifically, an orderly chemical grading in another tissue-tumor system besides that of liver, if found, would also show by comparing the two systems, whether the two kinds of high grade tumors were more alike than their parent tissues. This possibility is represented by any two lines in the subsidiary second version (dashed lines) in Fig. 1.

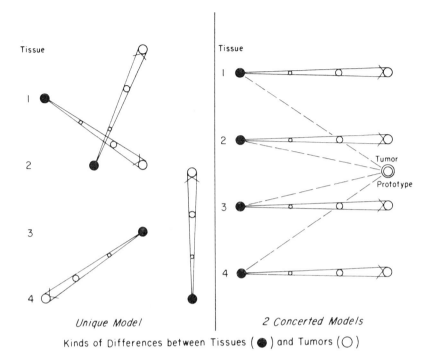

Tissue

Tissue

1

2

3

4

1

2

3

4

Tumor

Prototype

Unique Model

2 Concerted Models

Kinds of Differences between Tissues (●) and Tumors (○)

Fig. 1. *Alternative conceptual schemes of the relations between neoplasms and their tissues of origin, based on the accepted histological classification system.* Average differences between tissues and tumors show as distances on the map, in directions related to the kinds of differences. Individual normal tissues (●) are connected through increasing grades of their neoplasms to the most undifferentiated tumors (O). In the left-hand, "unique" model, the tumors each bear unique directional relations to their normal tissue of origin. In the right-hand, "concerted" model, all tumors differ in the same direction from normal tissues. A specialized version of the latter scheme (---) shows no distinctions remaining between the most undifferentiated tumors from all sources ("prototypic tumor").

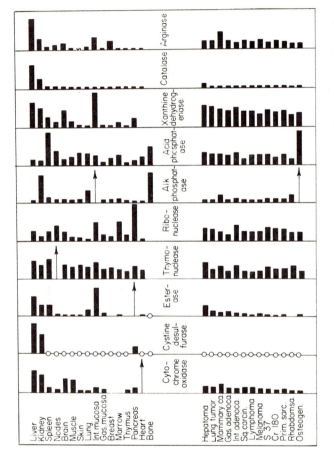

Fig. 2. *Relative enzyme activities in normal and neoplastic tissues of mice.* Lengths of horizontal bars in a column represent levels of a given enzyme (From Greenstein (3)).

50

Chemical Characterization of Neoplasia

It is possible to construct experimentally a map of the relations among tissues such as that diagrammed in Fig. 1. Average chemical differences between two tissues represent distance on the map. Examples of this have been published (2,6) and the mathematical techniques are widely used in other fields (7,8). The main needs are analyses of a sufficient number of components in every tissue to be compared. Systematic analyses of even single tissues are almost unknown in biochemistry, because its work has been partitioned among different tissues, ages, sexes and species of animals. Obviously, the quantitative analyses must be reliable and reproducible. Because enzymes characterize uniquely both the composition and function of tissues, they are the components of choice for such comparisons. There is more confusion than there ought to be in the minds of some biochemists about the validity of assays of enzymes in tissues by catalytic activity under standardized conditions. However, measurements of relative enzyme concentrations in different tissues can be reproduced in any laboratory using any adequate assay of that enzyme (9,10). The results are therefore accumulatable, and this will lessen the cost and increase the range of subsequent studies.

A careful selection of tissues and tumors is necessary to show the significant relationships with an utmost economy of analyses, because even the minimum number of analyses is a prodigious task. Transplanted tumors of the liver and mammary gland were chosen that represented in each case a spectrum of grades according to morphology and growth rate. Three different states of the mammary gland itself were analyzed because of uncertainty about which (virgin, pregnant and lactating glands) should be considered the tissue of origin of tumors. The results, surprisingly enough, turned out to be almost unaffected by the state of the gland. A number of other normal, adult and fetal tissues were subsequently analyzed to provide a background against which to view the tissues and tumors of primary interest.

A simpler preliminary study was encouraging (6). A random selection of enzymes with robust quantitative assays were measured. The amounts of 21 enzyme components in the critical tissues and tumors showed the chemical relationships among the tissues of the liver-hepatoma series and the mammary gland-mammary carcinoma series to be as indicated by dashed lines in Fig. 1. That is, undifferentiated

51

tumors from the two organs were very similar, differentiated tumors were less similar, and the two parent tissues were unlike (6).

We have since increased to 30 the number of components analyzed, included other normal tissues in the comparison, checked many of the analyses, and refined the numerical analysis (by the use of the logarithmic distribution among tissues of the values for a component and by the use of principal component analysis (11)). These were conservative modifications that provided a rigorous and objective test of the similarities initially found. The main differences between tissues in the latest study are graphed as distances in Fig. 3. The agreement with the subsidiary conceptual structure shown by dashed lines in Fig. 1 is close enough so that other alternatives for these two kinds of tumors can now be abandoned. The gradation, from left to right, of liver, slow- and fast-growing hepatomas confirms the monotonic relation within this series that has been repeatedly established by studies of one or a few components at a time to a total of well over a hundred substances (2). Some components are invariant in this series, but others either decrease or increase monotonically from liver to undifferentiated hepatomas (4). There is a similar gradation from left to right of mammary gland, differentiated and undifferentiated mammary carcinomas. It is not limited to hepatic tissues that chemical compositions of tumors change in parallel with loss of differentiation and increase of growth rate. Furthermore, the direction of gradation in both series means that the same general kinds of chemical changes occur in the different tumors. Finally, the two tissues of origin are chemically very different, but the tumors are less so. The highest grade tumors of the two kinds are very alike.

Relationships between tissues shown in Fig. 3 are remarkably stable. Half as many components give the same relationships and almost the same distances. The vertical and horizontal dimensions in Fig. 3 represent the two major ways in which two dozen rat tissues and tumors differ from one another. Each dimension encompasses a combination of analytical chemical values, and the components affecting one dimension more than the other can be ascertained. The vertical dimension distinguishes between normal adult tissues. Other such tissues besides liver and mammary gland are widely distributed in the vertical dimension, and are also to the left of the figure. Other kinds of tumors are more or less narrowly focused to the right of the figure.

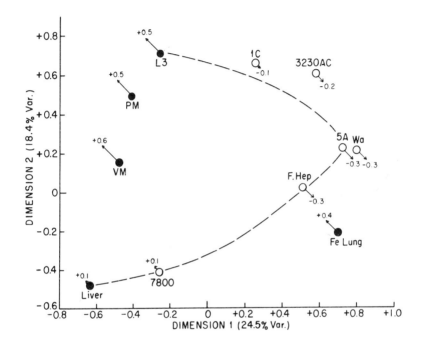

Fig. 3. *The kinds and amounts of the main chemical differences between normal rat tissues (●) and tumors (○).* The two dimensions (small arrows indicate the less important third dimension) from a principal component analysis of 30 components measured in twenty-four tissues account for nearly half of the variations between all tissues. Mammary glands (VM, virgin; PM, pregnancy; L3, third day of lactation) and mammary carcinomas (1C, 3230AC, 5A and Walker in order of increased dedifferentiation) are above the hepatic series of liver, slow-growing Morris hepatoma 7800, and fast-growing hepatomas (F. Hep.). Fetal lung (Fe Lung) is representative of most fetal tissues.

Fetal tissues are also narrowly distributed to the right of
Fig. 3 near the undifferentiated tumors. Fetal lung is
shown as representative of the cluster of fetal tissues that
surround it. Immature tissues (5 days after birth) are mid-
way to the adult tissues. The fetal tissues are closer together and therefore chemically resemble each other more
than do the adult tissues into which they differentiate, as
would be expected. They are near (*i.e.*, similar) to the
undifferentiated tumors, which also resemble each other
more than do the tissues from which they dedifferentiated.
Clearly, the horizontal dimension of Fig. 3 is an axis of
differentiation-undifferentiation. The most important components affecting location on this axis can also be identified. It is apparent that these chemical analyses show
meaningful interrelationships among tissues, and that selected analyses, such as those locating tumors toward the right,
could help distinguish between normal and cancerous tissues.

There can be no attempt to balance the chemical characterizations of these two tissue-tumor series in the rat
with the accumulated histological characterizations of all
tumors that now fill huge libraries. It is more to the
point that observations in another discipline, such as
chemistry, has quite readily confirmed the orderliness,
based on tissue cell type, that histologists created among
the welter of tumors they have examined. There are gradations between a normal tissue and its most undifferentiated
tumors that are confirmed by these independent observations.
So chemical measurements join morphological signs of dedifferentiation and anaplasia and the differences in behavior
such as growth rate as indicators of the greater or lesser
neoplastic character of a tumor. That there are such gradations is recognized by calling tumors "benign" or "malignant".
The fact can be stated more objectively and simply: there
are various degrees of neoplasticity among tumors of any
given kind. This is established histologically for at least
some kinds of tumors, and it is well-established biochemi-
cally for rat hepatomas. Perhaps now this scaled nature of
tumors should be recognized as a central and not a peripheral
characteristic of the phenomenon of neoplasia.

In addition, assuming that what has been shown for
these two kinds of experimental rat tumors is generally so,
the new chemical observations add to the resolution of
tumors from tissues in important ways. These are the relations between tumors of different kinds and between tumors
and immature tissues as shown in Fig. 3. Despite the chemi-

cal differences between various normal tissues, tumors of
these tissues differ from the parent tissues in much the
same chemical ways (*i.e.*, in the same direction in Fig. 3).
Although prescient pathologists have been aware of this
possibility, objective evidence for the "concerted" and
against the "unique" structures of a tumor classification
was lacking. Fig. 3 now points to an important unity among
neoplasms of all kinds. The unity shared by different kinds
of neoplasms consists of departures in the same direction
from normal and ending in a common type of tumor. The most
undifferentiated tumors from both tissues are so very similar that the existence of an "ideal" or prototype of tumor
composition is suggested. At the same time, the old paradox of similarity and diversity among tumors is resolved by
the varied degrees of differentiation of the tumors. More
differentiated tumors can be looked upon as greater or
lesser dilutions of the prototypic tumor with the composition of a particular normal tissue. Such admixture results
in closer similarity of a tumor to its own parent tissue,
greater chemical diversity between different kinds of tumors,
as well as moderation of a tumor to one that is less neoplastic in its behavior, form and composition.

The relationships between adult tissues and tumors that
were derived from studies of which Fig. 3 is only a part
can be represented diagrammatically as the surface of a
cone (Fig. 4). From the center of its base (more accurately
it is an indented base) the fetal tissues differentiate and
diverge to become the separate adult tissues along the rim
or conic perimeter. Tumors lie along the conic surface with
the least dedifferentiated ones close to the rim and the
most dedifferentiated ones at the apex. The latter are on
the axis with fetal tissues and not very far (not very
different) from them, since the indented base of this structure is more accurately a cone within the larger cone. Embryonic characteristics of tumors have often been noted,
and as often denied to be "truly" embryonic in character.
The objective chemical similarity of prototypic tumors to
embryonic tissues is, however, not unexpected. Although
fetal liver is more differentiated and less like prototypic
tumors (2) than most fetal rat tissues, Greenstein saw long
ago the chemical similarities of hepatomas to fetal liver
(1). Correlational analysis of his data confirmed his
conclusions (2: Chap. II). The relation to other fetal
tissues is closer. In merely logical terms, when the
specific chemical compositions that distinguish tissues are

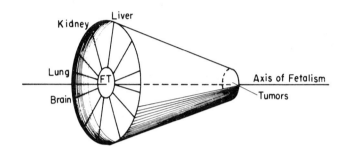

Fig. 4. *Geometric projection illustrating the relationships between tissues, with their average chemical differences expressed as distances.* Fetal tissues (FT) arise from the primordium at the hub of the wheel and diverge along the spokes into the differentiated adult tissues at the rim. A single tissue gives rise to a variety of tumors which can be arranged in order of loss of differentiation along the surface of the cone, and tumors from various tissues form series that converge toward the apex. The axis of the cone defines the most undifferentiated state of both normal and neoplastic tissues (From Knox (6)).

lost by tumors and they must move from the rim of the cone in Fig. 4, these *dedifferentiated* tumors could only come to resemble the still *undifferentiated* embryonic tissues.

Qualitative Chemical Similarities of Fetal and Tumor Tissues

Similarities between the quantitative patterns of components form the basis of the relationships between adult and fetal tissues and tumors shown in Figs. 3 and 4. Such a relation first emerged from intensive study of the liver-hepatoma series. Now it has been generalized to the mammary gland-mammary carcinoma series. The same sequence of hepatic and then other studies led to recognition of qualitative chemical characteristics which can specify the nature of tissues concretely. Observations on the occurrence of isozymes in hepatic tissues, often made in different laboratories, indicated that there was a rule governing the type of isozyme found in fetal and adult livers and in hepatomas (2: Chap. VIII). If fetal and adult rat livers had different forms of an enzyme, the fetal form was the one found in hepatomas. The only exceptions were rare and single occurrences of an adult isozyme in the most highly differentiated hepatomas. Some isozymes, like the M form of lactate dehydrogenase, occur in both fetal and adult livers, and in these cases, consistent with the rule, the same type of isozyme was also found in hepatomas. Subsequent work that was aimed specifically at testing this rule for liver and hepatomas has furnished us with additional examples (12). Following the sequence of study of hepatomas first, then of other tumors, it was important to know if the same rule held beyond the hepatomas. Could isozymes be identified in other immature tissues and were these replaced in the adult tissues, only to reappear in tumors of those same tissues?

Electrophoretic analyses of three isozyme systems were made in a number of rat tissues (Fig. 5). A particular form of each enzyme could indeed be recognized as the one predominating in all of the various fetal tissues examined. The same isozymic forms also predominated in tumors derived from liver, kidney, muscle and mammary gland (13). The forms of the three enzymes common to fetal and tumor tissues are listed in the lower half of Fig. 5. A different form of one or two of these enzymes predominated in each of the normal, adult tissues. These are enclosed in boxes in the upper half of Fig. 5.

57

PATTERNS OF THE PREDOMINANT ISOENZYMES
IN ADULT, FETAL AND NEOPLASTIC RAT TISSUES

	Liver	Kidney	Muscle	Mammary Gland
Adult Tissues				
LDH	M	H	M	M(H)
Aldolase	B	A(B)	A	A(C)
Pyruvate kinase	L	K	M	K
Fetal and Tumor Tissues				
LDH	M	M	M	M
Aldolase	A	A	A	A
Pyruvate kinase	K	K	K	K

Fig. 5. *Predominant isozymic forms of three enzymes found by electrophoresis in fetal, adult and tumor stages of four tissue systems.* Each isozyme is designated by a familiar letter. The identical patterns in fetal and tumor tissues are superimposed in the lower half of the table (no fetal version of mammary gland was examined). Boxes enclose the isozymes distinguishing differentiated (upperhalf) from undifferentiated states of a tissue (From Farron *et al*. (13)).

The results illustrate the same rule that holds for hepatomas, that these other immature and neoplastic tissues also share the same isozymes while the cognate adult tissues have at least some different forms. Investigation of still other enzyme systems should reveal more qualitative chemical evidences of differentiation in normal, growing tissues. Such isozymes would, perhaps, also be lost in tumors, and more such examples would increase the precision with which a tumor could be qualitatively distinguished. With only three enzymes, adult tissues showing rapid cell growth such as regenerating liver, small intestine and spleen had isozyme patterns only marginally different from that of fetal and tumor tissues.

Thus, like the quantitative comparisons, the qualitative chemical patterns of isozymes also show similarities between fetal and tumor tissues, and differences of both from adult tissues. The nature of the isozymes as specific proteins under genetic control allows a further conclusion about the tissue relationships. Certain parts of the genome that are active in mature tissues are turned off in tumors. Another part is activated. That part activated in tumors is normally active during tissue immaturity. In both immature and tumor tissues this part of the genome makes the same recognizable isozymes.

Chemical Distinctions of Tumors

A very large number of tissue components have had to be measured and identified in each of a number of fetal, adult and tumorous tissues to see the chemical relationships between these tissues. Still more assays will be needed to extend the findings to other tissue-tumor systems and to reveal, amongst the similarities, what particularly distinguishes tumors from normal tissues. Among the randomly chosen components needed in number to characterize each tissue, some, like those that move tumors to the right of adult tissues in Fig. 3, are of greater interest than others. Such components can be identified by the weights (factor scores) they have in each dimension of the factor analysis (11) from which Fig. 3 is derived. Specially interesting components can also be identified independently by stepwise discriminant analysis (11). This is a statistical technique that seeks to classify the tissues correctly into groups using the fewest possible components. The results can be graphed to show the degree of separation between group means and the dispersion of the groups. Seventeen normal (adult and fetal) tissues and seven tumors, among which those in Fig. 3 are included, can be separated in a significant manner by using only four of the thirty components that were measured. The separation of the two groups and the dispersion of the individual tissues within each group are shown in Fig. 6. The four enzymes which allow this clear distinction between normal and tumorous tissues happen to be the most efficient for this purpose among the thirty measured components. They are not otherwise remarkable, and doubtlessly still other components can be found that are as good or better discriminants, especially if particular isozymes are examined for this task. Fig. 4 does demonstrate, however, that there are usable chemical differences between sizable groups of normal and neoplastic tissues as was implied by the structures of Fig. 3. The separation is all the more remarkable because of the similarity of fetal to tumor tissues. It was therefore of interest to attempt to distinguish all three groups of adult, fetal and tumor tissues. This required only five enzyme measurements for a significant separation. It is shown in Fig. 7. Some of the enzymes used are common to Figs. 6 and 7. In general, relative abundance in certain tissues of each component may have a complex role of tightening one group or separating two groups. The method offers a way to screen out certain components for more detailed study of their contributions to the different natures of normal and neoplastic tissues.

Discussion

A new genre of biochemical investigations was necessary to gain the perspective shown here of the relations between rat tissues. Qualitative analyses have previously sufficed to construct metabolic maps showing the chemical unity of living systems. Quantitative comparisons of the catalytic activity of an enzyme within a laboratory have allowed many of them to be purified, and have permitted the regulation of their relative concentrations in a tissue to be studied. Now qualitative identifications and relative quantifications of enzymes in each of a series of tissues show the large variations on the theme of chemical unity that can be found among tissues that function differently. The individual enzymic patterns reflect these varied functions because of an intimate relation that exists between an enzyme and a

cell's activity. Enzyme analyses are measurements of the
things by which cells differ. The analyses are meaningful
because they can be reproduced in other laboratories and
fitted to cell functions. The results can be accumulated,
corroborated and their implications reexamined. Systematic
analyses of many tissues are needed in addition to the few
rat tissues described here. This can only be accomplished
by cooperative work in many laboratories. The preliminary
results indicate that the effort will be worthwhile.

Cooperative biochemical work related to cancer in many
laboratories over the past decade has focused on the rat
hepatomas, and specifically those graded in neoplasticity
between the extremes of adult liver itself and undifferentiated, fast-growing hepatomas. Given Greenstein's summary
that all tumors were similar, it was essential that the
chemical variety to be found among tumors of a single tissue
be demonstrated. The huge success of this inquiry may be
overlooked by failure in the ostensible goals of that cooperative effort (14): to detect some minimal deviation
among the normal variations of liver that would epitomize
cancerousness, and to do so by ignoring the full-blown devi-
ations that are plain and obvious in the highest grade
tumors. Preoccupation with minimal changes from the normal
crumbles as a strategy when a second kind of normal tissue
is investigated. What tumors of two tissues do have in
common are those characteristics shared by tumors regardless
of origin and that appear most recognizably in the "progressed", undifferentiated prototypic tumors. Disinterest in
the most "progressed" and altered tumors has caused them to
be overlooked as the reference standard for neoplasticity
in its purest form. This is what the prototypic tumor appears to be. Differentiated tumors appear to be diluted
versions of that prototype, diluted by the composition of
one or another normal tissue in the tumor series corresponding to that respective tissue.

The interpretations of these biochemical results draw
notable support from their parallel with the general histological description of neoplasms. Both approaches are
immeasurably strengthened by this concordance. The biochemical results have also extended or made more precise
some classical histological views by demonstrating the
similarity of undifferentiated tumors from two sources, by
recognizing the histological grades as steps in the series
culminating in a prototypic kind of tumor, and by furnish-
ing objective evidence for the long suspected relation be-

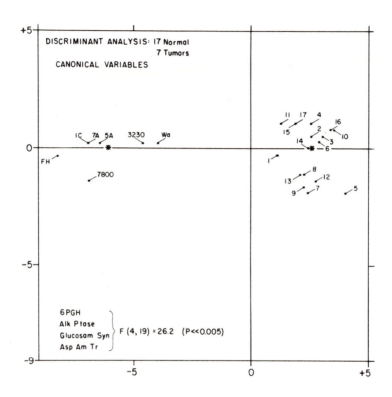

Fig. 6. *Statistically significant distinctions between groups of normal and neoplastic rat tissues made by discrimination analysis (11).* Tissue contents of the listed enzymes provided these separations (F-value is given) between the group of normal fetal and adult tissues (indicated by numbers at right) and the group of mammary carcinomas and hepatomas (labels at left), each about a group mean (*).

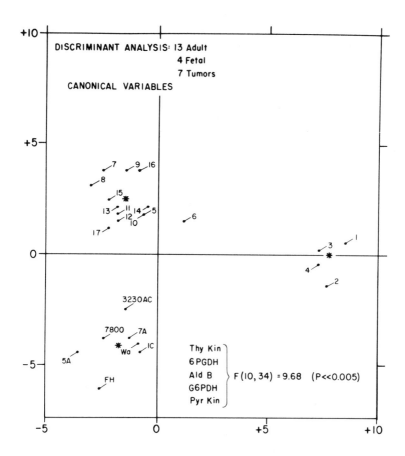

Fig. 7. *Statistically significant distinctions of the three groups of fetal, adult and tumor tissues.* Same analysis as Fig. 6. The fetal tissues (1-4) are liver, kidney, brain and lung, respectively.

tween tumors and normal, immature tissues.

This biochemical description of tumors is based upon their enzymic elements. Enzymes are intimately connected in one direction to the function of the cell, and in the other direction to the qualitative and quantitative expressions of the cell's genome. In these two directions, toward the biological nature of tumors and toward the genesis and regulation of them, are central areas of our ignorance of the cancer problem. Beyond the task of deepening and extending the chemical relationships between tissues and tumors that has been outlined here, we must address new formulations of old problems lying in both directions. Looking toward the biological nature of tumors, it would be helpful to design diagnostic and therapeutic modalities with the characteristics of the prototypic tumor in mind. In the other direction, we must learn what keeps one specific part of the genome active in an adult tissue, so that its state of differentiation is maintained. Future studies, necessarily including immature tissues as controls, should reveal the salient differences between the normal and abnormal undifferentiated tissues.

Summary

Analyses of the characteristic constituents (*e.g.*, the relative amounts of enzymic components) of rat tissues and tumors have been used to measure the degrees of chemical similarity among the tissues. Undifferentiated, fast-growing tumors originating from the liver and from mammary gland have almost the same compositions. Differentiated tumors from the same sources are more unlike in compositions, each kind tending to resemble the chemically very different parent tissues. A prototypic composition of tumors, whatever the source, appears to exist. When this is diluted by the various compositions of normal tissues, the products are tumors of lesser neoplastic character (more differentiated, slower growing, less autonomous tumors).

The prototypic composition of tumors is very similar, but not identical to that of many fetal tissues in both the quantitative patterns of enzymes and in the qualitative identities of certain isozymes. It appears that a fraction of the cell's genome acts in the same way in immature and tumorous tissues, but differently in adult tissues. Measurement of selected enzymes that are part, or are not part, of the prototypic composition of tumors can distinguish a variety of tumors from a variety of normal tissues. Relatively small numbers of enzymes (4 or 5) are sufficient to make this important distinction between the 24 normal and tumorous tissues examined.

A certain orderliness is now evident among the natures of tumors studied. Methods like those used here can focus attention upon the chemical components and processes that contribute most relevantly to the nature of neoplasms.

Presented by W. Eugene Knox. Supported by U.S. Atomic Energy Commission Contract AT(11-1)-3085 with the New England Deaconess Hospital and U.S. Public Health Service Grant AM 00567 and Research Career Award AM-K6-2018 from the National Institute of Arthritis, Metabolism and Digestive Diseases.

References

1. Greenstein, J.P. Biochemistry of Cancer, 2nd Ed., Academic Press, New York (1954).
2. Knox, W.E. Enzyme Patterns in Fetal, Adult and Neoplastic Rat Tissues, Karger, Basel (1972).
3. Greenstein, J.P. Some biochemical characteristics of morphologically separable cancers. Cancer Res. 16: 641-653 (1956).
4. Weber, G. and M.A. Lea. The molecular correlation concept of neoplasia. Advan. Enzyme Regulation 4: 115-145 (1966).
5. Weber, G. Molecular correlation concept: Ordered pattern of gene expression in neoplasia. Gann Monogr. 13: 47-77 (1972).
6. Knox, W.E. The protoplasmic patterns of tissues and tumors. Amer. Sci. 60: 480-488 (1972).
7. Sokal, R.R. and P.H.A. Sneath. Principles of Numerical Taxonomy, Freeman, San Francisco (1963).
8. Romney, A.K., R.N. Shepard and S.B. Nerlove. Multidimensional Scaling, 2 Vols., Seminar Press, New York (1972).
9. Mezl, V.A. and W.E. Knox. Comparison of two methods for the assay of glycogen phosphorylase in tissue homogenates. Enzyme 13: 197-202 (1972).

10. Schweitzer, E.S., F. Farron and W.E. Knox. Distribution of lactate dehydrogenase and its subunits in rat tissues and tumors. Enzyme 14;173-182 (1972-1973).
11. Dixon, W.J. BMD Biomedical Computor Programs, University of California Press, Berkeley (1970).
12. Weinhouse, S. Chapter 7, this conference.
13. Farron, F., H.H.T. Hsu and W.E. Knox. Fetal-type isoenzymes in hepatic and nonhepatic rat tumors. Cancer Res. 32: 302-308 (1972).
14. Wu, C. "Minimal deviation" hepatomas: A critical review of the terminology, including a commentary on the correlation of enzyme activity with growth rate of hepatomas. J. Nat. Cancer Inst. 39: 1149-1154 (1967).

CORRELATION BETWEEN CYCLIC AMP LEVELS AND MORPHOLOGICAL TRANSFORMATION INDUCED BY HOST OR VIRAL MUTATION

Richard A. Carchman

Introduction

Cyclic AMP has been postulated as a second messenger in the action of many hormones in eukaryotic cells (1) and as a regulator of transcription in *E. Coli* of the "lac" and "gal" operons (2,3). Furthermore, cAMP has also been shown to play an important role in controlling various properties of cultured fibroblasts (4-15). There are many factors which control the behavior of cultured cells, several of these also alter cAMP levels (16). cAMP has been shown to be involved in the regulation of the cell cycle (9), growth rate (7,8,12,13), saturation density (6), morphology (2,4,6,17), adhesion to the substratum (10), and the synthesis of mucopolysaccharides (14) and collagen (15). Various transformed cells have been shown to have low levels of cAMP when compared to their untransformed parent cells (8,18,19). Transformed cells have a more rapid growth rate, decreased adhesiveness and mucopolysaccharide synthesis, and increased agglutinability and an abnormal cellular morphology. These aberrant characteristics can be returned to near normal following treatment with DBcAMP or agents which raise cAMP levels (4,5,20). Therefore, these observations lend support to the proposal that many properties of transformed cells are due to their low levels of cAMP. This conclusion makes it appear likely that changes in cAMP metabolism play an important role in the transformation process.

Several of the questions we asked were: (1) Are cAMP levels related to an initial event in transformation and/or the maintenance of the transformed state? (2) How is its cellular concentration modified? (3) Can factors which modulate cAMP metabolism and transformation be isolated?

67

Materials and Methods

Table 1 lists all the cell lines used in this study; cells were routinely plated at 1×10^5 cells/dish and fed every other day. All cells were maintained in 5% CO_2, 95% air in 100% humidity at various temperatures. Cyclic AMP was measured in unwashed cells using the method of Steiner *et al.* (21) as modified by D'Armiento *et al.* (22). Nucleic acid was determined as described by Otten *et al.* (8). Adenylate cyclase and cyclic phosphodiesterase activity was measured according to previously described methods (23,24). Protein was determined by the method of Lowry using bovine serum albumin as the standard (25). Cell counts were determined using and Electrozone/celloscope by Particle Data Inc.

Results

Evidence has been accumulated, that in several different established contact inhibited cell lines, cAMP levels rise at confluency (8). There are reports in the literature, however, that at least in one cell line this was not observed (7). Table 2 shows the growth of NRK cells and it also shows the cAMP levels and the ratio between adenylate cyclase and phosphodiesterase (PDE) activities. Initially AC and PDE/ concomitantly rise, following confluency AC continues to rise, whereas PDE activity levels off. These cells are contact inhibited and reach a final saturation density of 20×10^6 cells/100 mm dish. As previously observed with 3T3 mouse embryo fibroblasts and WI 38 human diploid fibro-blasts (8), a close correlation exists between the growth rate of NRK cells and their cAMP levels. Cells growing in a logarithmic manner have low levels of cAMP and the ratio of AC/PDE is constant. At confluency the growth rate decreases and cAMP levels and the AC/PDE ratio starts to rise dramati-cally (Table 2). NRK cells clearly exhibit density dependent inhibition of growth, raise their cAMP levels at confluency, and the ratio of AC/PDE changes in a predictable fashion. CEF that have been maintained in culture beyond the second passage lose their ability to slow growth at confluency; they continue to grow until they slough off the plate. Their cAMP levels fail to rise, and the adenylate cyclase phospho-diesterase ratio does not change at confluency. The high degree of correlation between contact inhibition of growth

TABLE 1

Cell Lines

Cell Line	Additions	References
NRK	MSV	(36,37,38)
CEF	BH − Ta S−R − wt	(30,31,32)
	− wt T5	(39)
3T3/Balb	SV−40	(34,35)
3T3−4	Acridine dyes or spontaneous	(33)

NRK − Normal Rat Kidney

MSV − Murine Sarcoma Virus

CEF − Chicken Embryionic Fibroblasts

BH − Bryan High Titer − Rouse Sarcoma Virus

wt − wild type

Ta − Temperature Sensitive

S−R − Schmidt Ruppin

T5 − Temperature Sensitive

TABLE 2

NRK Cell Growth

[a]No. of Cells per plate x 10^6	MG Protein per plate	cAMP pMoles/MG Protein	AC/PDE[b]
DAYS			
3	1.5	0.33	8.7	4.2
5	12	2.32	6.5	3.8
7	15	3.4	13.2	6.5
11	22	4.5	34.4	18
12	20	4.8	39	

[a]Cells were counted on a Data Particle Counter

[b]Ratio of adenylate cyclase activity and cyclic phospho-diesterase activity.
cAMP formed/min/mg protein/cAMP hydrolysed/min/mg protein.
Substrate concentration 2mm ATP (AC) and 18 µM cAMP (PDE).

Cells were plated at 1 x 10^5/100 mm dish, maintained at 37°C and fed every 48 hours. They were fed the day before they were extracted for cAMP assay.

and rising cAMP levels as seen in NRK cells, and the fact
that in normal non-contact inhibited cells cAMP fails to
rise at confluency, strengthen the idea that cAMP is intimately involved in contact inhibition of growth.

One of the most useful tools available to answer some
of the questions we have posed is by using a normal cell
transformed by a temperature sensitive transforming virus.
At the permissive temperature the transformed phenotype
is evident. Recently Anderson *et al*. (26) have shown that
CEF cells infected with a RSV (BHWT) have lower levels of
adenylate cyclase activity than normal CEF. Using a temperature sensitive mutant of this virus it was demonstrated
that at the non-permissive temperature adenylate cyclase,
the enzyme responsible for cAMP synthesis is remarkably
similar to the enzyme in normal CEF. Within 10 min. of
shifting these cells to the permissive temperature, adenylate cyclase activity is decreased and is reduced two fold
within one half hour. Kinetic analysis of the enzyme
indicate quite clearly a change in the Km ATP and an altered response to increasing Mg^{++} concentration in the Km Mg^{++}.
The rapidity with which the transformed phenotype and the
fall in adenylate cyclase are seen after a shift to the
permissive temperature lead these authors to conclude that
a temperature sensitive viral product is directly responsible for these changes.

We have also looked at another transforming virus in
CEF. The Schmidt-Ruppin (SR) strain of RSV is another
transforming virus that alters cellular morphology, growth
and lowers cAMP levels. Unlike the adenylate cyclase in
the Bryan High Titer transformed cells, the S-R CEF cyclase
shows no altered affinity for ATP or Mg^{++} though it does
have a lower Vmax. A temperature sensitive mutant of this
virus has an additional mechanism for controlling its cellular cAMP levels. Following a shift to the permissive
temperature the S-R-Ts CEF extrude cAMP into the medium.
Therefore, in two different RSV infected cells, though
the cellular mechanisms for controlling cAMP metabolism are
strikingly different, the end result is the same, *e.g.* lower
cAMP levels and the transformed phenotype.

The infection of NRK cells with a MSV (Kirsten-non
producer strain) transforms these cells resulting in an
altered morphology and loss of contact inhibition of growth,
and cAMP levels fail to rise at confluency in these
transformed NRK cells. The addition of DBcAMP to these

71

cells returns their morphology toward normal and slows their
growth rate. The infection of NRK cells with a temperature
sensitive mutant of the K-MSV (t-6) results in a normal
cellular phenotype at 40°; these cells exhibit density dependent inhibition of growth and do not grow in soft agar.
Futhermore cAMP levels rise as growth slows in these cells
as they do in the NRK's (Table 3). Shifting the t-6 cells
to the permissive temperature (32°) does not produce any
clear morphologic change within 24 hr., nor do cAMP levels
change though they fail to rise as they do in the t-6 cells
at 40° (Table 4). T-6 cells shifted to 32° for several days
show the transformed phenotype, and their cAMP levels approach those of the t-6 cells maintained at 32° (Table 4) or
the KNRK cells grown at either temperature (Table 3), and
they are able to grow in soft agar. An analysis of how
cAMP metabolism is modulated by the cell under the above
conditions is currently underway. Hopefully these results
will help elucidate, in an established cell line, the
cellular control of cAMP in normal and transformed cells.

We have presented evidence in CEF infected with a
temperature sensitive RSV (RNA virus) that under permissive
and non-permissive conditions the active viral transforming
factor is present only at the permissive temperature where
altered morphology and low levels of cAMP are observed
even though virus is being produced at both temperatures.
In addition, similar effects were seen in an established
cell line (NRK) infected with another temperature sensitive
RNA virus (MSV), except that no virus is produced at either
the permissive or non-permissive temperature though the
viral transformation factor is active only at the permissive
temperature. In these two different systems the production
of virus itself is not essential to produce the transforming
effect.

We then looked at the effects of a DNA virus in a non-
permissive (non-transforming, non lytic system) cell line,
on cAMP levels and DNA synthesis. Simian Virus - 40 (SV-40)
is a member of the papova virus family. It is a small DNA
virus containing enough genetic information to code for
approximately six proteins (27). Confluent 3T3 cells were
exposed to a low input multiplicity of virus. At various
times after exposure to this virus cAMP levels were determined (Table 5). Parallel plates were analyzed for DNA
synthesis by radioautography (Table 5). Plates which were
untouched, mock infected, or exposed to UV-irradiated virus

TABLE 3

cAMP Levels and Growth

		Nucleic Acid				
		0.1	0.15	0.2	0.3	0.35
Growth Temperature						
NRK	32°	60^a	60	75	90	130
	40°	80	110	180		
KNRK	32°	30	30	30	40	35
	40°	35	30	35	35	35
T6	32°	35	35	35	30	30
	40°	80	85	90	110	120

a cAMP pMoles/mg Nucleic Acid

Cells were plated at 1 x 10^5 cells/60 mm dish at 32°C and fed every 48 hours. Some cells were then shifted and maintained at 40°C.

TABLE 4

Effects of Temperature Shift on cAMP Levels

Days		1	2	3
	40°	80	–	90
NRK	32°	80	–	78
	40°-32°	80	–	78
	40°	30	–	40
KNRK	32°	30	35	40
	40°-32°	30	40	37
	40°	70	88	84
TS6	32°	30	30	30
	40°-32°	70	70	40

[a] cAMP pMoles/mg Nucleic Acid

Cells were grown at 32°C, some were shifted to 40°C for several days and then shifted to 32°C.

TABLE 5

cAMP Levels and DNA Synthesis

Inoculum	Hours									% labeled nuclei
	1/2	1	2	3	4	6	8	10	11	
SV 40	90±1[a],[b]	-	75±(5.3)	50±(5.7)	50±(6)	50±(4.2)	80±(4.5)	80±(6)	80±(10)	16
Ultra Violet Irradiated SV 40	82±(1)	-	--	95±(1.3)	85±(5.7)	80±(4.5)	100±(6)	--	100±(6)	3
Sham Infected + 15% Serum	65	45	35	--	--	--	80	80	--	49

[a] % of untreated plates, each point is the mean of these percentages. Figures in parenthesis are standard error for each point.

[b] The average cAMP value for cells which were untouched is 49±3 pMoles/mg nucleic acid.

showed no change in cAMP levels or DNA synthesis (Table 5).
Whereas those cells exposed to Sv-40 virus had lowered cAMP
levels within 2-4 hours, reaching minimum levels in about
6 hours. Over the next 4-5 hours cAMP levels had returned
to near normal values. Autoradiography indicated a wave of
cellular DNA synthesis 18 hours after infection. We also
tested serum, an agent known to stimulate growth and lower
cAMP levels (16). As seen in Table 5, serum rapidly lowers
cAMP levels and increases DNA synthesis. The decrease in
cAMP levels produced by SV-40 in 3T3 cells is the earliest
known effect of the virus. The 2-4 hour lag period after
infection may represent the time for the virus to uncoat
and integrate with the cell genome. We are currently
examining this system in an attempt to identify the viral
product responsible for transformation and the decrease in
cAMP levels.

There is considerable data to indicate that low levels
of cAMP may be responsible for many properties of transformed cells, but there are some properties of transformed cells
which apparently are not under cAMP control. Recently we
have isolated host cell mutants which are defective in cAMP
metabolism. Adhesion to the substratum is a property of
cells which is very sensitive to cAMP. We selected for
host cell mutants that which exhibited a temperature sensitive change in adhesion.

The characteristic changes observed in these cells
after they are shifted from 39° to 23° for 10 min. are
clearly seen in Fig. 1. When the cells are maintained at
39°, cAMP levels are similar to the parent line. Within a
few minutes after shifting the mutant cell to 23° cAMP
levels decrease by 50%, whereas they are unchanged in the
parent cells (Table 6). This decrease in cAMP following
the temperature shift can be accounted for by its release
into the medium (Table 6). Within 5-10 min. after the
temperature shift the cell can be readily removed from the
plate by spraying the dish with medium from a pipette. By
15 min. 40-50% of the cells have retracted their processes
and have rounded up. Treating these cells with agents that
mimic or raise cAMP levels blocks the morphologic response
to the temperature shift (Table 6). Following a temperature shift, the cAMP levels are only transiently decreased;
then they begin to rise and overshoot and after 3-4 hours
are back to normal. Two other cellular properties are
closely associated with this change in cAMP levels: 1) the
cells flatten out and firmly adhere to the substratum,

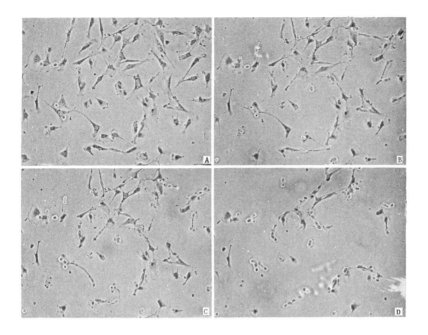

Fig. 1. *Morphology of 3T3cAMP^{ts}-1 cells after temperature shift or medium change.* A flask containing 3T3cAMP[ts]-1 cells in Dulbecco's modified Eagle's medium with 10% calf serum was maintained at a growth temperature of 39^5 °C. The flask was removed from the incubator and a selected field was photographed at 100 magnification in an inverted phase contrast microscope at room temperature within one minute (A). Photographs of this same field were taken without moving the flask on the microscope stage 5(B) and 10(C) minutes later. These demonstrate retraction of cell processes and rounding of individual cells. At this point many (20-50%) of the cells have disattached and could be removed by gentle agitation, but instead, the medium was gently poured off without agitation and new medium containing fresh 10% calf serum was added. Ten minutes later, another picture of this field was taken (D) showing even further (almost 100%) cellular rounding. Without medium change, the rounding would not have progressed much beyond the general amount seen in (C) (as measured by parallel experiments not shown).

TABLE 6

Effects of Temperature Shift on cAMP Levels

Treatment	3T3		Ts-1	
	Cells	Medium	Cells	Medium
None	42 ± 2.1^{a}	292^{d}	41 ± 2	116
Temperature Shift (10 min) (39.5^{o} to 23°C)	43 ± 1.7	306	20 ± 0.5	326
10% Calf Serum (cs)	–	–	26	–
10% CS + Temperature Shift (10 min)	–	–	19	–
PGE_1^{b} (prostaglandin E_1)	80	–	122	–
PGE_1^{c} + Temperature Shift (10 min)	86	–	160	–

[a] cAMP pMoles/mg nucleic acid

[b] PGE_1 $30\mu g/ml$ - 15 min.

[c] PGE_1 $30\mu g/ml$ - 15 min. before temperature shift

[d] Each point represents the amount of cAMP in two $50cm^2$

(dishes of cells containing 800 µg nucleic acid [pMoles])

2) they are refractory to a further temperature shift for 3-4 hours. These studies strongly indicate that cell shape and adherence of normal fibroblasts are regulated by cAMP.

Discussion

In light of studies on normal and transformed cells it is evident that the control of cAMP metabolism plays an integral role in modulating cell growth, morphology, adhesion, motility, agglutinability and mucopolysaccharide synthesis. The introduction of transforming virus to a cell results in the production of viral factors which may alter the plasma membrane, which in turn may depress adenylate cyclase activity, and coordinately effect other functions that are not dependent upon cAMP levels (6,28,29). Adenylate cyclase is closely associated with the plasma membrane and its activity is dependent on its membraneous milieu. Different viruses probably produce different transforming factors that interact with the cell in various ways, resulting in a decrease in adenylate cyclase activity. This decrease in AC activity may represent a pivotal event in the transformation of cells in culture. It is of great importance to clarify the nature of these viral factors in order to understand the question of cellular transformation.

Presented by Richard A. Carchman

References

1. Robison, G.A., R.W. Butcher, E.W. Sutherland. "Cyclic AMP". Academic Press, New York and London (1971).
2. Varmus, H.E., R. Perlman and I. Pastan. Regulation of "lac" messenger ribonucleic acid synthesis by cyclic adenosine 3',5' monophosphate and glucose. J. Biol. Chem. 245: 2259-2267 (1970).
3. Nissely, S.P., W.B. Anderson, M. Gottesman, R.L. Perlman and I. Pastan. *In vitro* transcription of the "gal" operon requires cyclic AMP and cyclic AMP receptor protein. J. Biol. Chem. 246: 4671-4678 (1971).
4. Hsie, A.W. and T.T. Puck. Morphological transformation of Chinese hamster cells by dibutyryl adenosine cyclic

3',5' monophosphate and testosterone. Proc. Nat. Acad. Sci. USA 68: 358-361 (1971).

5. Johnson, G.S., R.M. Friedman and I. Pastan. Restoration of several morphological characteristics of normal fibroblasts in sarcoma cells treated with adenosine 3',5' cyclic monophosphate and its derivates. Proc. Nat. Acad. Sci. USA 68: 425-429 (1971).

6. Johnson, G.S. and I. Pastan. Role of 3',5' Adenosine monophosphate in regulation of morphology and growth of transformed and normal fibroblasts. J. Nat. Cancer Inst. 48: 1377-1378 (1972).

7. Sheppard, J.R. Difference in the cyclic adenosine 3'5' monophosphate levels in normal and transformed cells. Nature New Biol. 236: 14-16 (1972).

8. Otten, J., G.S. Johnson and I. Pastan. Cyclic AMP levels in fibroblasts: Relationship to growth rate and contact inhibition of growth. Biochem. Biophys. Res. Commun. 44: 1192-1198 (1972).

9. Willingham, M.C., G.S. Johnson and I. Pastan. Control of DNA synthesis and mitosis in 3T3 cells by cyclic AMP. Biochem. Biophys. Res. Commun. 48: 743-748 (1972).

10. Johnson, G.S. and I. Pastan. Cyclic AMP increases the adhesion of fibroblasts to substratum. Nature New Biol. 236: 247-249 (1972).

11. Johnson, G.S., W.D. Morgan and I. Pastan. Regulation of cell motility by cyclic AMP. Nature 235: 54-56 (1972).

12. Bürk, R.R. Reduced adenyl cyclase activity in a polyoma virus transformed cell line. Nature 219: 1272-1275 (1958).

13. Ryan, W.L. and M.L. Heidrick. Inhibition of cell growth *in vitro* by adenosine 3',5' monophosphate. Science 162: 1484-1485 (1968).

14. Goggins, J.F., G.S. Johnson and I. Pastan. The effect of dibutyryl cyclic adenosine monophosphate on synthesis of sulfated mucopolysaccharides by transformed fibroblasts. J. Biol. Chem. 247: 5759-5764 (1972).

15. Hsie, A.W., C. Jones and T.T. Puck. Further changes in differentiation state accompanying the conversion of Chinese hamster cells to fibroblastic form by dibutyryl adenosine cyclic 3',5' monophosphate and hormones. Proc. Nat. Acad. Sci. USA 68: 1648-1652 (1971).

16. Otten, J., G.S. Johnson and I. Pastan. Regulation of cell growth by cyclic adenosine 3',5' monophosphate. J. Biol. Chem. 247: 7082-7087 (1972).

17. Johnson, G.S., R.M. Friedman and I. Pastan. Cyclic AMP treated sarcoma cells acquire several morphological characteristics of normal fibroblasts. Ann. New York Acad. Sci. 185: 413-416 (1971).
18. Granner, D., L.R. Chase, G.D. Auerbach and G.M. Tomkins. Tyrosine amino transferase: Enzyme induction independent of adenosine 3',5' monophosphate. Science 162: 1018-1020 (1968).
19. Heidrick, M.L. and W.L. Ryan. Adenosine 3',5' cyclic monophosphate and contact inhibition. Cancer Res. 31: 1313-1315 (1971).
20. Sheppard, J.R. Restoration of contact-inhibited growth to transformed cells by dibutyryl adenosine 3',5' cyclic monophosphate. Proc. Nat. Acad. Sci. USA 68: 1316-1320 (1971).
21. Steiner, A.L., C.W. Parker and D. Kipnis. Radioimmunoassay for cyclic nucleotides. J. Biol. Chem. 247: 1106-1113 (1972).
22. D'Armiento, M., G.S. Johnson and I. Pastan. Cyclic AMP and growth of fibroblasts: Effect of environmental pH. Nature New Biol. 242: 78-80 (1973).
23. Krishna, G., B. Weiss and B.B. Brodie. A simple sensitive method for the assay of adenyl cyclase. J. Pharmacol. Exp. Ther. 163: 379-385 (1968).
24. Brooker, G., L.J. Thomas and M.M. Appleman. The assay of adenosine 3',5' cyclic monophosphate and guanosine 3',5' cyclic monophosphate in biological materials by enzymatic radioisotopic displacement. Biochem. 7: 4177-4 (1968).
25. Lowry, O.H., N.J. Rosebrough, A.L. Farr and R.J. Randall. Protein measurement with the folin phenol reagent. J. Biol. Chem. 193: 265-275 (1951).
26. Anderson, W.B., G.S. Johnson and I. Pastan. Transformation of chick-embryo fibroblasts by wild-type and temperature-sensitive Rous Sarcoma Virus alters adenylate cyclase activity. Proc. Nat. Acad. Sci. USA 70: 1055-1059 (1973).
27. Eckhart, W. Onocogenic viruses. Ann. Rev. Biochem. 41: 503-516 (1972).
28. Gazdar, A., H. Masakazu, E. Russell and Y. Ikowa. Effects of dibutyryl cyclic adenosine phosphate plus theophylline on Murine Sarcoma Virus transformed non-producer cells (36930). Proc. Soc. Exp. Biol. Med. 141: 1044-1050 (1972).

RICHARD A. CARCHMAN

29. Sakiyama, H. and P.W. Robbins. The effect of dibutyryl
    adenosine 3',5' cyclic monophosphate on the synthesis
    of glycolipids by normal and transformed nil cells.
    Arch. Biochem. Biophys. 154: 407-414 (1973).
30. Nakata, Y. and J.P. Bader. Studies on the fixation
    and development of cellular transformation by Rous
    Sarcoma Virus. Virology 36: 401-410 (1968).
31. Bader, J.P. and N.R. Brown. Induction of mutations in
    an RNA tumour virus by an analogue of a DNA precursor.
    Nature New Biol. 234: 11-12 (1971).
32. Otten, J., J.P. Bader, G.S. Johnson and I. Pastan. A
    mutation in a Rous Sarcoma Virus gene that controls
    adenosine 3',5' monophosphate levels and transformation.
    J. Biol. Chem. 247: 1632-1633 (1972).
33. Peck, P.M., R.K. Preston and H.J. Creech. Mono and
    difunctional analogs of some quinoline and acridine
    nitrogen mustards. J. Org. Chem. 26: 3409-2414 (1961).
34. Jainchill, J. and G.J. Todaro. Stimulation of cell
    growth *in vitro* by serum with and without growth
    factor. Exp. Cell Res. 59: 137-146 (1970).
35. Kit, S., D.R. Dubbs, L.J. Piekaeski, R.A. de Tarres
    and J.L. Melnick. Acquistion of enzyme function by
    mouse kidney cells abortively infected with Papo-
    virus SV40. Proc. Nat. Acad. Sci. USA 56: 463-470
    (1966).
36. Duc-NGuYen, H., E.N. Rosenblum and R.F. Zeigel.
    Persistent infection of a rat kidney cell line with
    Rauscher Murine Leukemia Virus. J. Bacteriol. 92:
    1133-1138 (1966).
37. Rowe, W.P., W.E. Pugh and J.W. Hartley. Plaque assay
    techniques for Murine Leukemia Viruses. Virology 42:
    1136-1138 (1970).
38. Scolnick E.M. and W.P. Parks. Isolation and character-
    ization of a Primate Sarcoma Virus: Mechanism of
    rescue. Int'l. J. of Cancer (July, 1973, in press).
39. Martin G.S., M. Weber Venuta and H. Rubin. Tempera-
    ture-dependent alterations in sugar transport in cells
    infected by a temperature-sensitive mutant of Rous
    Sarcoma Virus. Proc. Nat. Acad. Sci. USA 68: 2739-
    2741 (1971).

82

CONTROL OF tRNA METHYLTRANSFERASE ACTIVITY BY COMPETING
ENZYME SYSTEMS

Sylvia J. Kerr

Introduction

The tRNA methyltransferases constitute a family of
enzymes which modify the structure of preformed tRNA by the
addition of methyl groups at the macromolecular level (1).
The study of the species specific methylating enzymes, which
confer structural and conformational individuality on tRNA
molecules is useful in understanding the complex interactions
in which tRNA is involved. Specific tRNA species and tRNA,
in general, play an essential role in regulation at a variety of levels in the cell including transcription (2), translation (3-7) and expression of enzyme activity (8-10).
    It has been established in a number of instances that
modulation of tRNA structure affects the functioning of this
molecule in protein synthesis in terms of amino acid acceptance (11), codon response (12), wobble (13) and ribosomal
binding (14-16) as well as its function in repression of
transcription (2), and alteration in the tRNA methyltransferases have been observed in many biological systems which
are being subject to shifts in regulatory mechanisms (Table
1) as well as in every tumor examined (17).
    Several investigators have reported differences in the
level of methylating enzymes in organs of foetal, newborn
and adult animals (21-24). We have discovered that these
differences are due in part to competing enzyme systems,
present in normal adult tissues and absent or present only
in low concentrations in foetal and tumor tissues, which
inhibit the tRNA methyltransferases by a dual mechanism, by
competition for substrate as well as by differential sensitivity to product inhibition (40). We report here on one such
system.

TABLE 1

Modulations of tRNA Methyltransferases in Biological Systems

System	References
Bacteriophage infection and induction	(18,19)
Insect metamorphosis	(20)
Embryonic vs. neonatal tissue	(21-24)
Colonizing slime mold	(25)
Differentiating lens tissue	(26)
Mammary epithelial cell differentiation	(27)
Ovariectomized uterus	(28,29)
Thyroxine-induced morphogenesis in the tadpole	(30)
Sea urchin embryogenesis	(31)
Germination of spores	(32)
Hormone-induced phosvitin synthesis	(33)
Phytohemagglutinin induction of lymphocytes	(34)
Viral transformation	(35,36)
Vitamin A and D deficient bone	(37)
Senescent tissues	(38,39)

Methods

Assays for tRNA methyltransferase and glycine N-methyl-transferase activity were carried out according to previously published procedures (40). S-Adenosylhomocysteine hydro-lase was assayed in the synthetic direction by determination of the disappearance of free sulfhydryl groups with Ellman's reagent, 5,5-dithiobis(2-nitrobenzoic acid). The incubation mixture contained 10 mM adenosine, 1 mM L-homocysteine, 50 mM Tris-HCl (pH 8.5), 1 mM EDTA and varying amounts of enzyme extract in a total volume of 0.2 ml. The reaction was stopped by addition of an equal volume of 10% TCA. The mixture was centrifuged and aliquots were taken for sulf-hydryl determination.

Results and Discussion

In Figure 1 comparisons of tRNA methyltransferase activity in extracts of liver from foetal, newborn and adult rabbit as well as in extracts from foetal and adult rabbit brain are presented. The extracts from foetal liver had a fourfold greater capacity to methylate tRNA than the extract from adult liver. Extracts of foetal brain tissue had a methylating capacity more than twice as great as the extract from adult brain. The decrease of enzyme activity beyond a certain concentration of protein in the case of the extracts from adult liver and brain implied the possible presence of an inhibitor in these extracts. Indeed, mixing experiments showed that the adult extracts could lower the methyltrans-ferase activity of the foetal extracts.

A separation of the tRNA methyltransferase activity and the inhibitory activity could be achieved because we have observed that at pH 5 the tRNA methyltransferase activity was essentially precipitated, while the inhibitor was found to remain in the supernatant (24). This simple separation permitted a study of the properties of the inhibitor.

The reneutralized pH 5 supernatant was inhibitory to tRNA methyltransferases from both adult and foetal organs. It was sensitive to heat and trypsin and lost its inhibitory activity upon dialysis. Filtration on Sephadex G-25 revealed that both a protein fraction and a low-molecular weight component were required for inhibition. The requisite low-molecular weight component was identified as glycine and the

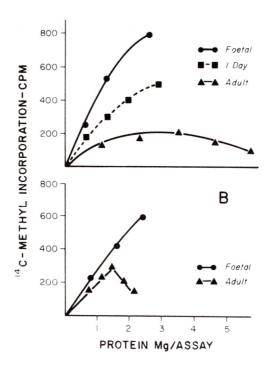

Fig. 1. *Methylation of tRNA by extracts from foetal, newborn and adult rabbit tissues.* Incubation was for 30 mins. at 37°. (A) Methylation by extracts from –10 day foetal, 1 day and mature rabbit liver. (B) Methylation by extracts from –10 day foetal and mature rabbit brain.

protein proved to be an enzyme which N-methylates glycine
to yield sarcosine (40).

The glycine N-methyltransferase from rabbit liver has
been purified to homogeneity using hydroxylapatite chromatography (41). The enzyme has a molecular weight of 123,500
as determined by sedimentation equilibrium centrifugation
and consists of 3 to 4 nonidentical subunits with molecular
weights in the range of 27,000 to 33,000 as determined by
mobility in sodium dodecylsulfate polyacrylamide gels. It
is a glycoprotein containing carbohydrate in the form of
sialic acid, 4 residues per mole of protein, and hexose,
2 residues per mole of protein, as well as 12 acetyl groups
per mole of protein. The amino-terminal group of the
protein is blocked.

In adult rabbit liver the glycine N-methyltransferase
represents from 0.9% to 3% of the soluble protein, and thus
is present in much higher concentrations than the tRNA methyltransferases. The relative specific activities of the
glycine N-methyltransferase and the tRNA methyltransferases
in crude extracts (Table 4) are such that the glycine
N-methyltransferase competes for all the available common
substrate, S-adenosylmethionine. However, when diluted in
an *in vitro* enzyme reaction, so that adequate S-adenosylmethionine remained for tRNA methyltransferase activity,
the tRNA methyltransferases were still inhibited. This
was traced to differential sensitivity to product inhibition
by S-adenosylhomocysteine as illustrated in Fig. 2. It can
be seen that at concentrations of S-adenosylhomocysteine
which barely affect the activity of the glycine N-methyltransferase, the tRNA methyltransferases are strongly
inhibited. The Michaelis-Menten affinity constants and
inhibitor constants for the two enzymes are presented in
Table 2.

The subcellular distribution of the two methyltransferase systems has been examined. After aqueous extraction
of tissues both enzymes are commonly found as soluble enzymes
in the 100,000 x g supernatant fluid. It has been reported,
however, that by the use of strictly nonaqueous fractionation techniques, the tRNA methyltransferases are found to be
primarily in the nuclear fraction (42). Rat liver nuclei,
prepared by nonaqueous extraction (42), were assayed for the
two methyltransferases and the results are summarized in
Table 3. It is evident that appreciable quantities of both
enzyme systems were present in the nuclear preparation and
in a ratio similar to that observed in aqueous cytoplasm.

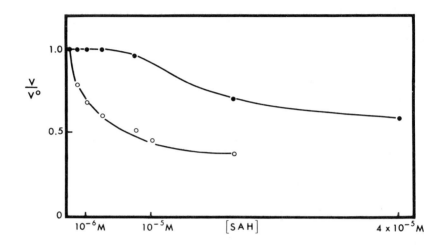

Fig. 2. *Inhibition of the tRNA methyltransferases and glycine methyltransferase from rabbit liver by S-adenosylhomocysteine (SAH).* (●—●) Glycine methyltransferase activity in the presence of 10^{-2} M glycine, 10^{-5} M S-adenosylmethionine and increasing concentrations of S-adenosylhomocysteine. (o—o) tRNA methyltransferase activity in the presence of 50 μg of tRNA and 10^{-5} M S-adenosylmethionine. Rates are expressed as percent of the initial reaction velocity (Vo) in the absence of added S-adenosylhomocysteine.

TABLE 2

Affinity and Inhibitor Constants of tRNA
Methyltransferase and Glycine Methyltransferase[a]

Enzyme	Km (SAM)[b]	Ki (SAH)[b]
tRNA methyltransferase	1.0 μM	2.0 μM
Glycine N-methyltransferase	100 μM	35 μM

[a]Values were derived from Lineweaver-Burk plots of kinetic
experiments. Lines were fitted to the points by the
method of least squares. Purified glycine methyltransferase
and pH 5 precipitated tRNA methyltransferases from adult
rabbit liver were used.

[b]Abbreviations are: SAM, S-adenosyl-L-methionine; SAH,
S-adenosyl-L-homocysteine.

TABLE 3

Relative Specific Activities of Glycine
Methyltransferase and tRNA Methytransferase in
Nuclear and Cytoplasmic Fractions from Rat Liver[a]

Enzyme source	Specific activity		Ratio of specific activity of glycine methyltransferase to specific activity of tRNA methyltransferase
	tRNA Methyltransferase	Glycine methyltransferase	
Nonaqueous nuclei	0.041	92.7	2260
Aqueous cytoplasm	0.046	162	3520

[a]Nuclei were prepared nonaqueously by published procedures
(42). Specific activity is expressed as nmoles/mg protein/
30 mins.

Thus, the glycine methyltransferase is in the same general
location as the tRNA methyltransferases and could conceiv-
ably contribute S-adenosylhomocysteine to the micro-milieu
in vivo.

Foetal liver and a number of tumors, in which tRNA
methyltransferase activity is elevated, were examined for
glycine N-methyltransferase activity. Foetal rabbit liver
and slow growing hepatomas showed very low levels of the
glycine N-methyltransferease activity while it was not
detectable at all in fast-growing hepatomas. These results
are summarized in Table 4.

A survey of adult tissues revealed that glycine N-methyltransferase was present in detectable amounts only in liver,
kidney and pancreas. These are the organs which show
relatively elevated levels of S-adenosylmethionine synthesizing enzyme. Mudd *et al*. (43) have demonstrated that
liver, kidney and pancreas have higher levels of the
adenosyltransferase than other tissues, with the majority
of tissues having 3% to 12% of the activity found in liver.
Lombardini and Tallalay (44) have also shown that levels of
adenosyltransferase in tumors is about 5% of that found in
normal liver.

S-Adenosylmethionine is an obligatory compound in over
40 known transmethylation reactions (45). Thus, the
control of its synthesis and use, as well as the control of
the accumulation of S-adenosylhomocysteine, is an important
metabolic process. Tissue levels of S-adenosylmethionine
appear to fall in a narrow range of about 0.02 to 0.1 μmoles
per gram of wet weight tissue (46,47). No difference was
found in these levels in a number of solid rodent tumors
(44). There is one report, however, of elevated levels of
S-adenosylmethionine in leukemic white blood cells (48). In
that case the level in the leukemic cells was more than 4
times greater than the level found in normal white blood
cells. The physiological implications of this finding are
not clear. Levels of the S-adenosylmethionine synthesizing
enzyme in these preparations were not determined, but it has
been shown that the level of tRNA methyltransferase activity
is almost 10-fold greater in leukemic white blood cells than
in normal lymphocytes (49). What competing or regulatory
enzyme systems might be present in normal cells and absent
from the leukemic cells is not known.

Concentrations of S-adenosylhomocysteine have not been
as extensively investigated, but in mammalian liver it
appears to be present at a concentration of 0.06 to 0.07

91

Table 4

Distribution of Enzymes in Various Tissues[a]

Species	Tissue	tRNA methyl-transferase	Glycine N-methyl-transferase	S-adenosylhomo-cysteine hydrolase
		nmoles/mg/30 min	nmoles/mg/30 min	nmoles/mg/30 min
Rabbit	Foetal liver	0.023	12.8	180
	Liver	0.016	649	1300
	Pancreas	0.050	64.5	500
	Kidney	0.037	3.0_b	305
	Brain	0.038	N.D.[b]	90
Rat	Liver	0.018	135	970
	Morris hepatoma			
	9618A	0.023	1.8	380
	5123D	0.076	2.6_b	300
	3924A	0.051	N.D.[b]	114
	Novikoff hepatoma	0.353	N.D.[b]	200

[a]All assays were performed under standard conditions. The values are means derived from tissues of three individual animals. Female Holtzmann rats weighing 200 grams were used for control normal rat liver. Mature New Zealand white rabbits and -5 day foetal liver from the same species were used in the examination of rabbit tissues.

[b]Not detectable.

μmoles per gram wet weight (50); essentially in levels
equivalent to those of S-adenosylmethionine. It is apparent
that at physiological levels of these compounds, the activity
of the tRNA methyltransferases would be affected, while the
glycine N-methyltransferase activity would remain essentially
intact.

The main pathway in mammalian tissues for the degradation of S-adenosylhomocysteine is its enzymatic hydrolysis
to adenosine and L-homocysteine (51). This enzyme, S-adenosylhomocysteine hydrolase, then, is of importance in keeping
S-adenosylhomocysteine from building up to damaging inhibitory levels. We have assayed the hydrolase in a number of
tissues and the results are included in Table 4. It is
evident that in those organs with high levels of glycine
N-methyltransferase activity the S-adenosylhomocysteine
hydrolase activity is elevated in a parallel manner.

Another interesting aspect of the interrelation between
the tRNA methyltransferases and glycine N-methyltransferase
emerged from studies of the enzymes in aging tissues. An
inverse relationship was observed between the two enzymes
in such studies.

Between the age of 3 months and 12 months, the specific
activity of the glycine N-methyltransferase increases 30% in
rat liver while in rat kidney the increase is 40%. During
the same period the capacity of the tRNA methyltransferases
is lowered by 35% in the older animals (39). Coincidentally,
it has been reported that the S-adenosylmethionine synthesizing enzyme shows a 35% decrease in livers of older rats
(52).

Figures 3 and 4 demonstrate a similar increase in
glycine N-methyltransferase and decrease in tRNA methyltransferase activity between mature and senile mouse livers
(12 to 30 month livers). Whether such decreases in tRNA
methyltransferase activity lead to hypomethylation of tRNA,
with a possible decrease in functional fidelity, has not
yet been determined.

Another competing enzyme system which has been observed
in rat liver and human liver is nicotinamide N-methyltransferase (53-54). Upon addition of nicotinamide to crude
liver extracts tRNA methyltransferase activity is inhibited,
probably by a mechanism similar to that involved with
glycine N-methyltransferase. tRNA methyltransferases in
crude extracts from a number of rodent and human tumors are
also inhibited by addition of nicotinamide (55), indicating
that the nicotinamide methyltransferase is present in near

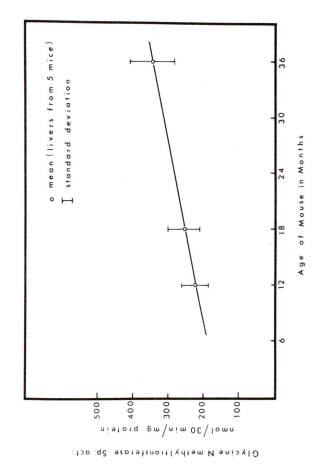

Fig. 3. *Glycine N-methyltransferase activity of C57 B1/6J male mouse liver.* Each point is the mean from two determinations on each of five mice (39).

94

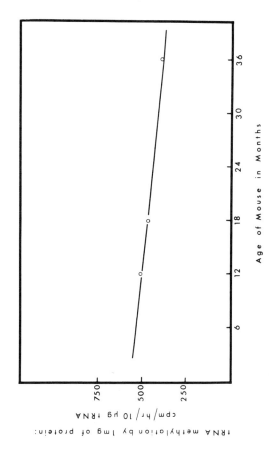

Fig. 4. *tRNA methyltransferase activity in C57 B1/6J male mouse liver.* Determinations were on the same animals as in Fig. 3 (39).

95

normal levels in the tumor tissues. This is contrary to
the glycine N-methyltransferase system, which is very low
or absent in a number of tumor tissues.

In organs which lack the glycine N-methyltransferases
there appear to be other competing enzyme systems which
affect their tRNA methyltransferase activity.

Swiatek *et al.* (56) have reported the appearance of an
inhibitor of the tRNA methyltransferases soon after birth
in pig brain. The system has not yet been characterized,
but may well represent a competing enzyme.

In an organ which is under hormonal control, the uterus,
changes in the tRNA methyltransferases have been observed in
response to estrogen (28,29). The enzyme level falls in the
uterus of an ovariectomized animal but can be restored to
normal levels by administration of physiological amounts of
estradiol. These alterations in tRNA methyltransferase
activity appear to be due to fluctuations in inhibitor
levels in the uterus. This is evidenced by the separation
by pH 5 precipitation of the tRNA methyltransferase from
the inhibitor, when as a result of the separation, the
levels of tRNA methyltransferase activity are equivalent
for ovariectomized and normal uteri.

Thus, it would appear that just as there is an organ
variation and specificity of the tRNA methyltransferases
(57), there is an organ variation in the regulatory mechanisms controlling these enzymes. It is not clear yet just
how this regulation affects the expression of these enzymes.
However, in many of the systems discussed here novel isoaccepting transfer RNA's have been observed. Foetal rabbit
liver contains four different isoaccepting tRNA species,
tRNA^{Arg}, tRNA^{Leu}, tRNA^{Lys}, and tRNA^{Met}, as compared to
adult rabbit liver (58). Altered tRNA's in aged mosquitos
have been reported (59), and deficient modification in the
tRNA^{Phe} of senescent wheat leaf has been detected (60).

It was also observed that in the ovariectomized
uterus a new tRNA^{Ser} appears which disappears after the
administration of physiological doses of the hormone (28).

All tumors examined have also shown variant isoaccepting tRNA's (17). Whether these variations in isoaccepting
tRNA species represent alterations in modification or in
primary sequence is yet to be determined.

The high tRNA methyltransferase capacity in tumor
tissues and the disappearance of competing enzyme systems
in these tissues may represent a derepressed state or an
expression of the total tRNA methyltransferase capacity of

the species, which is normally only expressed in foetal tissue. Other similarities between foetal and tumor tissues have been observed, such as the foetal antigens associated with some tumors (61), and, more pertinently, certain transfer RNA species found in tumor tissue, which have no counterparts in normal adult tissue but are present in foetal tissue (62-64).

Our understanding of cellular regulatory mechanisms will have to be extended before we can assign any function in differentiation or oncogenesis to the changes in tRNA modifying enzymes, inhibitors of these enzymes and tRNA's themselves observed in these systems.

Presented by Sylvia Kerr from the Department of Surgery, University of Colorado Medical Center, Denver, Colorado 80220. Supported in part by Research Grant CA-12742-01 from the National Cancer Institute and National Institutes of Health Contract 71-2186. The author is a Research Career Development Awardee of the National Cancer Institute, United States Public Health Service.

References

1. Borek, E. and P.R. Srinivasan. The methylation of nucleic acids. Ann. Rev. Biochem. 35: 275 (1966).
2. Singer, C.E., G.R. Smith, R. Cortese and B.N. Ames. Mutant tRNA^{His} ineffective in repression and lacking two pseudoridine modifications. Nature New Biol. 238: 72 (1972).
3. Marcker, K. The formation of N-formylmethionyl-sRNA. J. Mol. Biol. 14: 63 (1965).
4. Smith, J.D., J.N. Abelson, B.F. Clark, H.M. Goodman and S. Brenner. Studies on *amber* suppressor tRNA. Cold Spring Harbor Symp. Quant. Biol. 31: 479 (1966).
5. Carbon, J., P. Berg and C. Yanofsky. Missense suppression due to a genetically altered tRNA. Cold Spring Harbor Symp. Quant. Biol. 31: 489 (1966).
6. Anderson, W.F. and J.M. Gilbert. tRNA-dependent translational control of *in vitro* hemoglobin synthesis. Biochem. Biophys. Res. Commun. 36: 456 (1969).
7. Wainwright, S.D. Stimulation of hemoglobin synthesis in developing chick blastodisc blood islands by a minor

alanine-specific transfer RNA. Cancer Res. 31: 694
(1971).

8. Duda, E., M. Staub, P. Venetianer and G. Denes.
Interaction between phenylalanine-tRNA and the allosteric first enzyme of the aromatic amino acid biosynthetic pathway. Biochem. Biophys. Res. Commun. 32:
992 (1968).

9. Hatfield, G.W. and R.O. Burns. Specific binding of
leucyl transfer RNA to an immature form of L-threonine
deaminase: its implications in repression. Proc.
Nat. Acad. Sci. USA 66: 1027 (1970).

10. Jacobson, K.B. Role of an isoacceptor transfer ribonucleic acid as an enzyme inhibitor: effect on trpto-
phan pyrrolase of drosophila. Nature New Biol.
231: 17 (1971).

11. Shugart, L., G.D. Novelli and M.P. Stulberg. Isolation
and properties of undermethylated phenylalanine transfer RNA from a relaxed mutant of *Escherichia coli*.
Biochim. Biophys. Acta 157: 83 (1968).

12. Capra, J.D. and A. Peterkofsky. Effect of *in vitro*
methylation on the chromatographic and coding properties of methyl-deficient leucine transfer RNA. J.
Mol. Biol. 33: 591 (1968).

13. Yoshida, M., K. Takeishi and T. Ukita. Anticodon
structure of GAA-specific glutamic acid tRNA from
yeast. Biochem. Biophys. Res. Commun. 39: 852 (1970).

14. Fittler, F. and R.H. Hall. Selective modification of
yeast seryl tRNA and its effect on the acceptance and
binding functions. Biochem. Biophys. Res. Commun. 25:
441 (1966).

15. Thiebe, R. and H. Zachau. A specific modification
next to the anticodon of phenylalanine transfer
ribonucleic acid. Europ. J. Biochem. 5: 546 (1968).

16. Gefter, M.L. and R.L. Russell. Role of modifications
in tyrosine transfer RNA: a modified base affecting
ribosome binding. J. Mol. Biol. 39: 145 (1969).

17. Borek, E. and S.J. Kerr. Atypical transfer RNA's and
their origin in neoplastic cells. Advances in
Cancer Research 15: 163 (1972).

18. Wainfan, E., P.R. Srinivasan and E. Borek. Alterations
in the transfer ribonucleic acid methylases after
bacteriophage infection or induction. Biochem. 4
2845 (1965).

19. Wainfan, E., P.R. Srinivasan and E. Borek. Inhibition
of tRNA methylases in lysogenic organisms after

induction by ultraviolet light or heat. J. Mol. Biol.
22: 349 (1966).

20. Baliga, B.S., P.R. Srinivasan and E. Borek. Changes
in the tRNA methylating enzymes during insect metamorphosis. Nature 208: 555 (1965).

21. Kaye, A.M., B. Fridlender and R. Salomon. RNA methylase systems in various species and in normal and neoplastic organs. Israel J. Chem. 3: 78 (1965).

22. Hancock, R.L., P. McFarland and R.R. Fox. sRNA
methylase of embryonic liver. Experientia 23: 806
(1967).

23. Simon, L.N., A.J. Glasky and T.H. Rejal. Enzymes in
the central nervous system. I. RNA methylase.
Biochim. Biophys. Acta 142: 99 (1967).

24. Kerr, S.J. Natural inhibitors of the transfer ribonucleic acid methylases. Biochem. 9: 690 (1970).

25. Pillinger, D.J. and E. Borek. Transfer RNA methylases
during morphogenesis in the cellular slime mold. Proc.
Nat. Acad. Sci. USA 62: 1145 (1969).

26. Kerr, S.J. and Z. Dische. tRNA methylases in bovine
lens. Invest. Ophthalmol. 9: 286 (1970).

27. Turkington, R.W. Hormonal regulation of transfer
ribonucleic acid and transfer ribonucleic acid–methylating enzymes during development of the mouse mammary
gland. J. Biol. Chem. 244: 5140 (1969).

28. Sharma, O.K. and E. Borek. Hormonal effect on transfer ribonucleic acid methylases and on serine transfer
ribonucleic acid. Biochem. 9: 2507 (1970).

29. Sharma, O.K., S.J. Kerr, R. Lipshitz-Wiesner and E.
Borek. Regulation of the tRNA methylases. Federation
Proc. 30: 167 (1971).

30. Pillinger, D.J., E. Borek and W.K. Paik. tRNA methylases during thyroxine-induced differentiation in bull
frog tadpoles. J. Endocrinol. 49: 553 (1971).

31. Sharma, O.K., L.A. Loeb and E. Borek. Transfer RNA
methylases during sea urchin embryogenesis. Biochim.
Biophys. Acta 240: 558 (1971).

32. Wong, R.S.L., G.A. Scarborough and E. Borek. Transfer
ribonucleic acid methylases during germination of
Neurospora crassa. J. Bacteriol. 108: 446 (1971).

33. Mays, L.L. and E. Borek. Transfer ribonucleic acid
methyltransferases during hormone-induced synthesis of
phosvitin. Biochem. 10: 4949 (1971).

34. Riddick, D.H. and R.C. Gallo. Transfer RNA methylase
activities of human lymphocytes. I. Induction by

PHA (phytohemagglutinin) in normal lymphocytes. Blood 37: 282 (1971).

35. Kit, S., K. Nakajima and D.R. Dubbs. Transfer RNA methylase activities of SV-40 transformed cells and cells infected with animal viruses. Cancer Res. 30: 528 (1970).

36. Gallagher, R.E., R.C.Y. Ting and R.C. Gallo. Transfer RNA methylase alterations in polyoma transformed rat embryo culture cells. Proc. Soc. Exptl. Biol. Med. 136: 819 (1971).

37. Bradford, D.S., B. Hacker and I. Clark. Transfer ribonucleic acid methylases of bone. Studies on vitamin A and D deficiency. Biochem. J. 126: 1057 (1972).

38. Wust, C.J. and L. Rosen. Aminoacylation and methylation of tRNA as a function of age in the rat. Exp. Geront. 7: 331 (1972).

39. Mays, L.L., E. Borek and C.E. Finch. Glycine N-methyltransferase: A regulatory enzyme which increases in aging animals. Nature (in press).

40. Kerr, S.J. Competing methyltransferase systems. J. Biol. Chem. 247: 4248 (1972).

41. Heady, J.E. and S.J. Kerr. Purification and character-ization of glycine N-methyltransferase. J. Biol. Chem. 248: 69 (1973).

42. Kahle, P., P. Hoppe-Seyler and H. Kroger. Transfer RNA methylases from rat liver nuclei. Biochim. Biophys. Acta 240: 384 (1971).

43. Mudd, S.H., J.D. Finkelstein, F. Irrevere and L. Laster. Transsulfuration in mammals. J. Biol. Chem. 240: 4382 (1965).

44. Lombardini, J.B. and P. Talalay. Formation, functions and regulatory importance of S-adenosyl-L-methionine. Advances in Enzyme Regulation 9: 349 (1971).

45. Mudd, S.H. and G.L. Cantoni. Biological transmethyla-tion, methyl-group neogenesis and other "one-carbon" metabolic reactions dependent upon tetrahydrofolic acid. In: M. Florkin and E. Stotz (Editors). Comprehensive Biochemistry, Vol. 15, Elsevier, Amster-dam (1964), p. 1.

46. Baldessarini, R.J. and I.J. Kopin. S-adenosylmethionine in brain and other tissues. J. Neurochemistry 13: 769 (1966).

47. Baldessarini, R.J. Alterations in tissue levels of S-adenosylmethionine. Biochem. Pharmacol. 15: 741 (1966

48. Baldessarini, R.J. and P.P. Carbone. Adenosylmethionine elevation in leukemic white blood cells. Science 149: 644 (1965).
49. Tsutsui, E., P.R. Srinivasan and E. Borek. tRNA methylases in tumors of animal and human origin. Proc. Nat. Acad. Sci. USA 56: 1003 (1966).
50. Salvatore, F., V. Zappia and S.K. Shapiro. Quantitative analysis of S-adenosylhomocysteine in liver. Biochim. Biophys. Acta 158: 461 (1968).
51. de la Haba, G. and G.L. Cantoni. The enzymatic synthesis of S-adenosylhomocysteine from adenosine and homocysteine. J. Biol. Chem. 234: 603 (1959).
52. Finkelstein, J.D. Methionine metabolism in mammals. Effect of age, diet and hormones on three enzymes of the pathway in rat tissues. Arch. Biochem. Biophys. 122: 583 (1967).
53. Murai, J.T., P. Jenkinson, R.M. Halpern and R.A. Smith. The inhibition of tRNA methylase activity by nicotinamide and a non-dialyzable inhibitor. Biochem. Biophys. Res. Commun. 46: 999 (1972).
54. Kuchino, Y. and H. Endo. Nicotinamide and its methyltransferase as apparent inhibitors of tRNA methylase. J. Biochem. 71: 719 (1972).
55. Buch, L., D. Streeter, R.M. Halpern, L.N. Simon, M.G. Stout and R.A. Smith. Inhibition of transfer ribonucleic acid methylase activity from several human tumors by nicotinamide and nicotinamide analogs. Biochem. 11: 393 (1972).
56. Swiatek, K.R., D.G. Streeter and L.N. Simon. Transfer ribonucleic acid methylase activity in the developing pig brain. Biochem. 10: 2563 (1971).
57. Turkington, R.W. and M. Riddle. Transfer RNA-methylating enzymes in mammary carcinoma cells. Cancer Res. 30: 650 (1970).
58. Kerr, S.J. Differences in tRNA's in embryonic and adult liver. Federation Proc. 29: 893 Abs. (1970).
59. Hoffman, J.L. Quantitative and qualitative changes in mosquito tRNA as a function of age. Federation Proc. 31: 866 Abs. (1972).
60. Shugart, L.R. The inability of tRNA[Phe] from senescing tissue of wheat to participate in poly(U)-stimulated polyphenylalanine formation. Federation Proc. 30: 1271 Abs. (1971).
61. Gold, P. Antigenic reversion in human cancer. Ann. Rev. Med. 22: 85 (1971).

62. Holland, J.J., M.W. Taylor and C.A. Buck. Chromato-graphic differences between tyrosyl-tRNA from different mammalian cells. Proc. Nat. Acad. Sci. USA 58: 2437 (1967).

63. Yang, W.K. Isoaccepting transfer RNA's in mammalian differentiated cells and tumor tissues. Cancer Res. 31: 639 (1971).

64. Gonano, P., G. Pirro and S. Silvetti. Foetal liver tRNA^{Phe} in rat hepatoma. Nature New Biol. 242: 236 (1973).

PROPERTIES OF THYMIDINE KINASE ENZYMES ISOLATED FROM MITOCHONDRIAL AND CYTOSOL FRACTIONS OF NORMAL, BROMODEOXY-URIDINE-RESISTANT, AND VIRUS-INFECTED CELLS

Saul Kit, Wai-Choi Leung and David Trkula

Thymidine Kinase and the Pharmacological Effects of Thymidine Analogs

Thymidine (dT) kinase is a very interesting enzyme. It catalyzes the phosphorylation of dT, dU, and of halogenated analogs of dU [*e.g.*, dBU, dIU, dFU and 5-trifluoromethyl-2'-deoxyuridine (F_3dT)]. Thus, it is responsible for converting dFU and F_3dT, respectively, to dFUMP and 5'-trifluoromethyl-2'-deoxyuridylic acid, potent inhibitors of dTMP synthetase. However, by also catalyzing the phosphorylation of dT to dTMP, dT kinase provides an alternative pathway (the salvage pathway) for circumventing the drug-induced block of *de novo* dTMP synthesis. dT kinase activity is critical for the antitumor and antiviral effects of dFU, dBU and F_3dT (1,2). Indeed, the responsiveness of different transplantable mouse leukemias *in vivo* to dFU is inversely correlated with tumor cell levels of dT kinase (1).

By phosphorylating dBU, dT kinase initiates the reactions which enable dBU to be incorporated in place of dT into DNA. This substitution of dBU for dT in DNA increases the incidence of mutations (3), sensitizes DNA to photochemical damage (4), increases the buoyant density of DNA in CsCl equilibrium density gradients, and makes the DNA more stable to heat denaturation and less stable to alkaline denaturation (5,6). Based upon the photosensitivity of dBU-containing DNA, Puck and Kao (7) developed an elegant method for selecting nutritionally-deficient mammalian cell mutants. Boettiger and Temin (8) employed the photosensitivity of dBU-DNA to show that the Rous sarcoma virus genome is converted to a DNA intermediate (provirus) during viral transformation of chick embryo fibroblasts. The distinctive physico-chemical properties of dBU-containing DNA have been used in numerous experiments on semiconserva-

tive and repair replication of DNA (9,10), to label the
initiation point and terminus of DNA replication (11), for
genetic mapping (12), and for demonstrating bidirectional
DNA replication (13).

Treatment of cells with dBU profoundly affects the
expression of cellular and viral genetic information and
cell differentiation. These effects are dT kinase-depen-
dent, since the incorporation of dBU into DNA is necessary
for dBU to have its effects, and the changes caused by dBU
can be reversed by dT.

Treatment of cells with dBU (or with dIU) activates
phage and SV40 formation, respectively, in lysogenic bacteria
and in SV40-transformed hamster cells (14,15). It activates
C-type virus production in virus-negative clones of high
leukemic AKR mouse cells (16), in low leukemic BALB/c cells
(17), in nonproducer mouse sarcoma virus transformed rat
cells (18,19), in mouse melanoma cells (20), and in established lines of human tumor cells (21). dBU-treatment also
induces Epstein-Barr virus synthesis in virus negative
lymphoid cells (22,23).

Low concentrations of dBU which do not interfere with
cell multiplication inhibit the expression of the following
differentiated functions: (a) the fusion of myoblasts to
form multinucleated myotubes and the synthesis by myoblasts
of myosin (24); (b) the sprouting of neurites by presumptive
neuroblasts; (c) the secretion of hyaluronic acid by amnion
cells; (d) and the synthesis of chondroitin sulfate by
chondrocytes (25-27). Enzymes engaged in chondroitin sulfate
synthesis are progressively inhibited by dBU treatment of
chondrocytes (26). Pigment formation is inhibited in retina
cells (28) and in mouse melanoma cells (20) and the tumorigenicity of the melanoma cells decreases while the immunogenicity increases. The synthesis of hyaluronic acid and
the activity of hyaluronate synthetase are reduced by dBU-
treatment of a somatic hybrid of mouse and Chinese hamster
cells (29). Dimethylsulfoxide (DMSO) treatment greatly
increases the synthesis of heme and of the α and β globin
chains of hemoglobin in Friend virus-induced leukemic cells.
dBU inhibits this DMSO-stimulated differentiation, while
enhancing the budding of Friend virus from the leukemic
cells (30). Mammary epithelial cell differentiation is
inhibited, as is the formation of casein and α-lactalbumin
(both induced by prolactin) (31). Synthesis of the adrenal
steroid inducible enzyme, tyrosine aminotransferase, is
dramatically reduced when an established line of rat

104

hepatoma cells is grown in culture with dBU (32). The effect is selective since the rates of cell growth and of general protein synthesis are relatively unaffected and the concentrations of several other enzymes are not changed.

The effects of substituting dBU for dT in DNA are probably mediated at the level of transcription. Jones and Dove (33) have shown that dBU-substitution in DNA reduces by seven-fold DNA-directed RNA production and sensitizes bacterial transcription capacity to near visible light irradiation. Lin and Riggs have suggested that altered binding of regulatory proteins may be the underlying mechanism of the dBU effect (34). They found that lac repressor binds 10-times tighter to dBU-substituted lac operator than it does to normal lac operator. If the simple presence of a repressor on the operator were sufficient to cause repression of transcription, then dBU substitution would render the induction of operons more difficult, *i.e.*, higher concentrations of inducer would be needed. To explain the activation of C-type viruses by dBU, they speculated that the altered binding of regulatory proteins results in the disruption of finely tuned regulatory systems that hold the viruses in check.

dT Kinase, DNA Synthesis and Growth

The synthesis and the activity of dT kinase is subject to complex physiological controls. dT kinase synthesis is inducible and induction of this enzyme is associated with DNA synthesis. dT kinase undergoes rapid turnover at a time when cells enter the stationary growth phase. Furthermore, the activity of dT kinase is subject to feed-back inhibition.

dT kinase is induced in cells infected with four classes of DNA-containing animal viruses (Table 1). The induction process requires new RNA and protein synthesis, occurs prior to the start of viral DNA replication, and can take place even if viral DNA synthesis is inhibited by drugs or ultraviolet (UV)-irradiation. Indeed, extended dT kinase synthesis is observed when cells are infected with UV-irradiated viruses or when cells are treated at the time of infection with inhibitors of DNA synthesis.

High enzyme levels are found in various human and animal tumors, in cell cultures transformed by oncogenic viruses, and in fetal tissues (Table 2). Among normal adult

TABLE 1

DNA-Containing Animal Viruses that Induce Thymidine Kinase[a]

Virus Group	Virus
Poxvirus	Vaccinia, rabbit pox, cowpox, ectromelia
Herpes virus	Herpes simplex types 1 and 2, pseudorabies
Adenovirus	Simian adenoviruses types 15 and 32
	Human adenoviruses types 2, 5 and 12
	Adenovirus 7-SV40 hybrid
Papovavirus	Polyoma, SV40

[a]*See:* S. Kit and D.R. Dubbs, ref. 75.

TABLE 2

Tissues and Physiological Conditions with Elevated dT Kinase Activities

System	Reference
Chorionic Gonadotrophin-stimulated large oocytes of *Xenopus laevis*	(35)
Isoproterenol-stimulated DNA synthesis in mouse salivary gland	(36)
Estrogen-induced, estrogen-dependent mammary and adrenocortical tumors of rats (maintained by estrogen pellets or prolactin)	(37,38)
ACTH-stimulated adrenals of guinea pigs	(39)
Growth hormone-stimulated adipose tissue of hypophysectomized rats	(40)
Wing epithelium of silkworm pupae during development (ecdysone)	(41)
Regenerating rat liver	(42-45)
Compensatory hypertrophy of rat kidney after unilateral nephrectomy	(46)
Rat fetal liver and spleen engaged in erythropoiesis	(47,48)
Proliferating adult rat tissues (bone marrow, thymus, spleen, small intestine)	(47)
Minimal deviation hepatomas, Novikoff and H-35 hepatomas *vs* adult liver	(49,50)
Human neoplastic *vs* matched normal tissues	(51)
Acute lymphocytic or granulocytic leukemia *vs* normal leukocytes	(52)
Developing breast muscle of dystrophic chickens	(53)
Germinating spores of *Bacillus subtilis*	(54)
Synchronous growth of *Physarum polycephalum*	(55,59)
Maximum at a defined stage of the cell cycle during synchronous division of fertilized sea urchin eggs	(56)

tissues, dT kinase activity is high in bone marrow, thymus, spleen, and small intestine, and low in kidney, brain, lung, pancreas, testes, and lactating mammary gland. dT kinase is induced during liver regeneration and in kidney undergoing compensatory hypertrophy. In 9 transplanted rat tumors (nonhepatic), there is a direct correlation between dT kinase content and growth rate (doubling time ranging from 1 to 23 days). In fetal rat liver, the enzyme has the highest activity between the seventeenth and nineteenth day of gestation. In rat spleen there is a striking rise after birth to values several times higher than in fetal or adult spleen. It is known that liver during fetal life and spleen during early postnatal life are temporary erythropoietic organs. Thus, both organs exhibit the highest dT kinase activities at a time when they are most active in erythropoiesis (47). All minimal deviation hepatomas show elevated levels of dT kinase compared with host liver. Sneider, Potter, and Morris have commented that the most consistent increase in enzyme activity in hepatomas is that of dT kinase (50). The failure of this enzyme to be repressed under conditions that repress its synthesis in normal adult liver cells may be the best indication of malignancy so far available in hepatomas. The consistent elevation in dT kinase is more striking (3 to 40-fold) than that for any other enzyme or enzyme system studied thus far, including glycolysis.

dT kinase is induced in tissues during hormonal-stimulated DNA synthesis. In the case of estrogen-induced, estrogen-dependent rat mammary and adrenocortical carcinomas, the tumors regress and dT kinase activity decreases significantly in 2 to 4 days after the estrogen pellets are removed from ovariectomized females. However, in the absence of estrogens, the kinase levels can be maintained by administering prolactin. Estrogen withdrawal does not cause a reduction of dT kinase activity in autonomous tumors (37,38).

During the administration of growth hormone to hypophysectomized rats, dT kinase activity increases slightly after 1 day, rises sharply to a maximum at 2 days, and then decreases to about half the maximal value by the fourth day. Stimulation of DNA synthesis by growth hormone follows the same temporal pattern. The increases in dT kinase and in DNA synthesis are both inhibited by cortisone (40).

At any time during the long period of diapause in silkworm pupae, injection of ecdysone or its secretion by the pupae's own thoracic glands provokes the initiation of adult development. Simultaneously, DNA synthesis and mitotic activity are resumed after months of developmental standstill and dT kinase activity increases 20-fold (41).

One characteristic of hereditary muscular dystrophy is an increased content of DNA in the dystrophic muscle. In chickens with hereditary muscular dystrophy, the DNA content of the pathological muscle, on a gram wet weight basis, is not only greater than that in corresponding controls over most of the life cycle investigated, but the patterns of change during late embryonic and early post-hatching development stages differ markedly. In control muscle, DNA content is at a maximum at day 18 of embryonic development and then declines to a base line value by 3 months after hatching. In the dystrophic muscle, DNA content is similar to control values at 18 days *in ovo*, but continues to increase to a maximum level about one week *ex ovo* and then decreases. Despite this decrease, DNA content of muscle from dystrophic chickens 1 to 6 months of age is still significantly greater than that in corresponding controls. These and other changes have led to the hypothesis that hereditary muscular dystrophy in the chicken represents a defect in normal maturation and development. It is thus significant that dT kinase levels are high during the period of myoblast cell division and DNA synthesis in normal chick embryos (up to day 12) and then decreases, but in dystrophic embryonic tissue, the decline in dT kinase is delayed until at least day 19 *in ovo*, which correlates with the continued increase in DNA content until after hatching and with a delay in myotube formation (53).

Very low dT kinase activity is found in crude extracts of *Bacillus subtilis* spores as compared with extracts from vegetative cells. dT kinase activity increases during spore germination simultaneously with the initiation of DNA synthesis. Increases in dT kinase activity are prevented by chloramphenicol, indicating that *de novo* protein synthesis is required. By delayed addition of chloramphenicol, dT kinase can be distinguished from early proteins synthesized during the first 30-80 min. after germination. Synthesis of dT kinase is controlled independently from DNA synthesis by the cellular mechanisms since, even when X-irradiation prevents DNA synthesis in the germinating spores, dT kinase is induced (54).

The addition of serum to confluent monolayer cell cultures can provoke a round of DNA synthesis and cell division. In the serum-treated cultures, dT kinase is enhanced from 10 to 20 hr. after treatment and this enhancement precedes the initiation of DNA synthesis. Arabinofuranosyl-cytosine (ara-C) treatment of the cultures at the time of serum addition prevents the initiation of DNA synthesis but enhances the stimulation of dT kinase activity (57).

In synchronized cultures of Chinese hamster fibroblasts, dT kinase activity is low in the G1 phase, rises during the S phase (the phase of DNA synthesis), remains high during G2 and mitosis, and decreases sharply again to low values when the cells postmitotically re-enter G1 (58). Periodic dT kinase production has also been observed in synchronous plasmodia of *Physarum polycephalum* (55,59), synchronous populations of HeLa cells (60), and during synchronous division of fertilized sea urchin eggs (56).

dT kinase turnover has been studied in cell cultures and in normal and regenerating rat liver. After LM mouse fibroblast cultures reach the stationary phase of the growth cycle, the total dT kinase activity per culture sharply declines and, concomitantly, the cultures display a greatly reduced capacity to incorporate ^{3}H-dT into cellular DNA (61). This decline can be delayed by treating cultures with dT, the substrate of dT kinase. From experiments in which stationary phase cultures were treated with puromycin to prevent protein synthesis, Kit, Dubbs and Frearson (61) estimated that the half life of dT kinase is about 3 hr. Bresnick, Williams, and Mosse (45) studied dT kinase turnover *in vivo* in normal and regenerating rat liver. Using cycloheximide and actinomycin D to analyze the turnover of the enzyme and its RNA template, they found that the turnover of dT kinase in control and regenerating rat liver was 2.6 hr. and 3.7 hr., respectively, and the turnover of the RNA template in control and regenerating rat liver was 3 hr. and 7 hr., respectively. The mechanisms determining dT kinase turnover are not understood. We are currently investigating the hypothesis that protease enzymes are involved in this turnover.

dT kinase activity is markedly inhibited by dTTP, the end product of the salvage pathway. The degree of inhibition by dTTP depends upon the ATP concentration. dT kinase activity is very unstable *in vitro*, but the activity can be stabilized by the substrates, dT and ATP, and by the end-product inhibitor, dTTP (61). The observation that the substrates stabilize dT kinase activity has been used to advantage during purification of the enzyme and for study of the enzyme during polyacrylamide gel electrophoresis and

110

glycerol gradient centrifugation.

dBU-Resistant, dT Kinase-Deficient Cell Lines

In 1963, Kit, *et al.* (62) adapted LM mouse fibroblast cells to grow in dBU containing media. Equilibrium density gradient centrifugation experiments demonstrated that these dBU-tolerant cells incorporated dBU in place of dT into chromosomal DNA. Additional lines of dBU-tolerant SV40-transformed mouse kidney (63) and malignant melanoma cells (64) have subsequently been obtained. In fact, a mutant Syrian hamster melanoma line with a growth dependence on dBU has recently been described by Davidson and Bick (65).

After prolonged subculture in high concentrations of dBU, LM mouse fibroblast cells developed increased resistance to dBU and their properties changed. Equilibrium density gradient centrifugation experiments then showed that the highly resistant cells, named LM(TK⁻), no longer incorporated dBU into chromosomal DNA. Isotope incorporation and radioautographic experiments also showed that the LM(TK⁻) cells and their clones (*e.g.*, clone 1D) did not incorporate ^{3}H-dT into cellular DNA. Growth experiments demonstrated that the cells were cross-resistant to dFU, dIU, and to dT concentrations which blocked the growth of normal cells. Furthermore, the cells were killed by aminopterin, even in media containing dT, hypoxanthine, and glycine (HATG medium).

To explain the properties of the dBU-resistant cells, it was postulated that they were deficient in dT kinase, the first enzyme in the metabolic pathway needed for the utilization of dT, dBU, and dFU. This was confirmed by direct enzyme analyses (62). Subsequently, additional lines of mutant mouse (65), human (66), Chinese hamster, and Syrian hamster (67) cells with dBU-resistance and a dT kinase deficiency were isolated.

Littlefield (68) and Davidson and Ephrussi (69) recognized that dBU-resistant cell lines could be very useful for selecting somatic cell hybrids. This could be accomplished by co-cultivating dBU-resistant cells with azaguanine resistant cells in HATG medium. The parental dBU-resistant and azaguanine-resistant lines lack dT kinase and hypoxanthine phosphoribosyl transferase, respectively, and hence, they are killed when the *de novo* pathways of dTMP and IMP synthesis are inhibited by aminopterin. However, the

somatic hybrids obtain the dT kinase and hypoxanthine phosphoribosyl transferase genes from each of their respective
parental lines and, thus, can utilize the dT and hypoxanthine in the HATG medium. They can therefore grow despite
the aminopterin inhibition of *de novo* biosynthetic pathways.

Numerous somatic cell hybrids have now been obtained
using drug-resistant cell lines and selective HATG medium
(67). The somatic hybrids have been employed to study the
role of genes in the regulation of cellular synthetic
activities, to study genetic complementation and linkage,
and for experiments in virology and oncology (70,71). For
example, using somatic hybrids of human and mouse cells,
Miller and collaborators (72) showed that the dT kinase
locus is on human chromosome 17. Green and coworkers (73)
developed a method for enriching a population of human-
mouse somatic hybrids for cells containing multiple copies
of the dT kinase chromosome. Harris and coworkers (74)
studied the suppression of malignancy in somatic hybrids
formed by fusing high with low malignant mouse lines.

LM(TK⁻) cells have been used in our laboratory to
demonstrate that herpes simplex type 1 and vaccinia viruses
induce virus-specific dT kinases in enzyme-deficient cells
(75). The dT kinases induced by vaccinia and herpes simplex
type 1 differ from host cell dT kinase in kinetic, electrophoretic and immunological properties. In addition, the
dT kinase induced by herpes simplex type 1 differs from the
enzymes induced by herpes simplex type 2 and pseudorabies
viruses (75-78). Using the LM(TK⁻) cells, mutant strains
of vaccinia and herpes simplex viruses, deficient in dT
kinase-inducing activity, were later isolated.

dBU-resistant, dT kinase-deficient hamster, mouse,
and human cell lines have also been used to investigate
the role of oncogenic virus genes in dT kinase induction.
It was shown that polyoma and human adenoviruses induce
dT kinase activity in enzyme-positive, but not in enzyme-
deficient cell lines (75,79). These results signify that
papova- and adenoviruses can turn on cellular dT kinase
synthesis, but do not themselves code for this enzyme.
Similarly, Moloney sarcoma-leukemia complex (MSV-MLV) does
not induce dT kinase in enzyme-deficient mKS (BU100) cells.
However, MSV-MLV infection of dT kinase-positive 3T3 cells
causes a delay in dT kinase turnover (Table 3). This
delayed turnover is associated with loss of contact inhibition and transformation of the cultures (80).

Recently, Munyon and coworkers (81) have shown that

112

TABLE 3

Thymidine (dT) Kinase Activity of Noninfected and MSV–MLV
Infected 3T3 (Mouse) Cells[a]

| | | dT Kinase Activity[b] | |
Experiment	Days PI	Noninfected	MSV–MLV-Infected
1	1	7.2	6.0
	2	11.0	5.0
	5	1.5	4.0
2	5	1.6	8.4
	8	0.1	2.5

[a]See reference (80). Cells were infected with MSV–MLV
24 hr. after seeding.

[b]Picomoles dUMP formed per µg protein in 10 min. at 38°.

infection of LM(TK⁻) cells with UV-irradiated herpes simplex virus causes a small portion of the cells (10^{-5}) to acquire the dT kinase-positive phenotype. This conversion process is associated with the acquisition by the cells of the herpes simplex-specific dT kinase (82). These observations gain significance from the demonstration by Duff and Rapp (83) that UV-irradiated herpes simplex viruses are capable of transforming hamster embryo cells to neoplasia.

Rothschild and Black (84) have suggested that the enzymes functioning in the dTTP-salvage pathway of DNA biosynthesis may have a regulatory role in promoting tumor formation. They isolated cells deficient in dT kinase from transplantable SV40-induced hamster tumors. When inoculated into hamsters, the dT kinase-deficient cells were less transplantable than parental, dT kinase-positive cells. Tumors which did arise from such cells had prolonged latent periods and contained a mixture of enzyme-positive and enzyme-deficient cells. Revertants contained intermediate dT kinase levels and displayed an oncogenic potential intermediate between the wild-type and the enzyme-deficient cells. dT kinase may not be required under growth conditions in culture where enriched media are supplied, but may become rate-limiting for growth under conditions prevailing in the body of an animal.

The Properties of HeLa(BU25) Cells

At this point, we would like to recall some of the properties of the HeLa(BU25) line of dT kinase-deficient human cells. Extracts of HeLa(BU25) cells are deficient in dU, dT and dBU phosphorylating activity (66). Growth of HeLa(BU25) cells is not inhibited by 25 µg/ml dBU and is only partly reduced by 100 µg/ml dBU. Radioautographic experiments have shown that after HeLa(BU25) cells are incubated with ^{3}H-dT or ^{3}H-dBU, fewer nuclei are labelled than with parental HeLa S3 cells, and the nuclei of the HeLa(BU25) cells are only lightly labelled. Density gradient centrifugation experiments of isolated nuclear DNA also show that HeLa(BU25) cells are deficient in the incorporation of exogenous dBU into nuclear DNA. The nuclear DNA of HeLa S3 bands in CsCl density gradients at a density of 1.696 g cm^{-3}. After 5 days of growth in dBU medium, the density of HeLa S3 DNA is increased to 1.753 g cm^{-3}. HeLa(BU25) cells have been propagated for over 61 passages

114

in medium containing 25 μg/ml dBU. In contrast to the
DNA of HeLa S3 cells, the nuclear DNA of HeLa(BU25) cells
exhibits a buoyant density of 1.700 g cm^{-3} even after the
cells are grown for 5 additional days in medium with 100 μg/
ml dBU (85). Thus, the nuclear DNA of HeLa(BU25) cells
does not become "heavy" due to the incorporation of dBU.

HeLa(BU25) cells fail to grow in HATG medium. Furthermore, human adenovirus type 5 (Ad 5) replication is grossly
inhibited in HeLa(BU25) cells in HATG medium (79). In
contrast, Ad 5 replicates normally in dT kinase-positive
KB cells in HATG medium and in either KB or HeLa(BU25) cells
in medium lacking aminopterin. This indicates that insuffici-
ent dTMP is generated from exogenous dT in HATG medium to
support the replication of Ad 5 in HeLa(BU25) cell nuclei.

Considering these properties of HeLa(BU25) cells, it
was surprising to find during studies of DNA synthesis that
HeLa(BU25) cells incorporate normal amounts of exogenous
^{3}H-dT into *mitochondrial* DNA (86). This observation
suggested that despite the loss of the principal dT-dU phosphorylating enzyme, HeLa(BU25) cells retain a mitochondrial
specific dT-dU phosphorylating enzyme. Studies with purified mitochondrial extracts demonstrated that this was
indeed the case. Clayton and Teplitz (87) and Attardi and
Attardi (88) have also demonstrated that dT kinase-deficient
LM(TK$^-$) clone 1D cells incorporate dBU into mitochondrial
DNA, although they do not incorporate dBU into nuclear DNA.
A genetically distinct dT kinase was detected in the mitochondria of LM(TK$^-$) clone 1D cells and in other lines of
dT kinase-deficient mouse cells (86,89,90).

A situation analogous to that observed in mutant
mammalian cells exists in algae. Several investigators have
shown with a variety of algal species that exogenous dT can
be incorporated into chloroplasts but not into nuclei. If
^{3}H-dTMP is supplied, radioactivity is incorporated into
both nuclear and cytoplasmic DNA in proportion to the
abundance of these DNA components. These observations
indicate that algae lack cytoplasmic dT kinase, but contain
a chloroplast-specific dT kinase (91).

Distribution of dT Kinase Activity in Parental and Mutant
Animal Cell Lines

Table 4 shows the relative distribution of dT kinase
in cytosol (post-microsomal high speed supernatant fraction)

TABLE 4

dT Kinase Activities of Cytosol and Mitochondrial Fractions[a]

Cell Line	Species	Cell Fraction	dT Kinase Activity per 10^6 Cells	% of Total Cytosol plus Mitochondrial dT Kinase Activity	Specific Activity[b]
LM	Mouse	Cytosol	19,000	98.9	16.2
		Mitochondria	200	1.1	0.4
LM(TK⁻)	Mouse	Cytosol	0	0	0
		Mitochondria	140	100	0.3
mKS-A	Mouse	Cytosol	29,000	99.7	11.2
		Mitochondria	85	0.3	0.1
mKS(BU100)	Mouse	Cytosol	0	0	0
		Mitochondria	67	100	0.1
HeLa S3	Human	Cytosol	56,300	96.9	11.1
		Mitochondria	1,830	3.1	1.6
HeLa(BU25)	Human	Cytosol	160	19.1	0.02
		Mitochondria	670	80.9	0.5
WI38 Va 13A	Human	Cytosol	95,800	97.3	23.0
		Mitochondria	2,710	2.7	2.3

[a]Mitochondrial and cytosol extracts were centrifuged for 1 hr. at 105,000 x g and high speed supernatant fractions assayed with ^{3}H-dU as nucleoside acceptor.
[b]Picomoles dUMP formed at 38°C per μg protein. Incubation time was 10 min. for HeLa S3, HeLa(BU25), and WI38 Va 13A cells, and 20 min. for all mouse lines.

and mitochondrial fractions of parental and enzyme-deficient human and mouse lines. In dT kinase-positive cell lines, small amounts of dT kinase activity were detected in the microsomal, nuclear, and mitochondrial fractions, but more than 95% of the total cellular activity was in the cytosol fraction. The specific activities of the cytosol dT kinases of enzyme-positive human and mouse lines, respectively, were 10-fold and 22-40 fold greater than that of the mitochondrial enzymes. In contrast, the mitochondrial dT kinase accounts for 81% of the total mitochondrial plus cytosol activity of HeLa(BU25) cells and for all of the activity of mutant mouse lines. The specific activities of the mitochondrial dT kinases of mutant cells were of the same order of magnitude as those from the mitochondria of parental cells.

Phosphate Donor Specificities and Feed-back Inhibitors

Two enzymes capable of catalyzing the phosphorylation of dT, dU, and dBU are known. In animal cells and in *E. coli*, the principal phosphorylating enzyme is dT kinase, an enzyme which uses ATP as phosphate donor and is subject to end-product inhibition by dTTP. This enzyme does not phosphorylate Urd, Cyd, or dCyd. In contrast, the enzyme catalyzing the phosphorylation of dT, dU, and dBU in *Clostridium perfringens*, *Tetrahymena pyriformis* and in various plant tissues is nucleoside phosphotransferase. Urd, Cyd, and dCyd are also phosphorylated by nucleoside phosphotransferase. The phosphotransferase uses various nucleoside mono-phosphates and diphosphates as phosphate donors and is not inhibited by dTTP. Nucleoside phosphotransferase activity has been detected in chick embryo, but not in rat embryo tissues.

In view of the postulated evolution of mitochondria from endosymbiotic bacteria (94), the hypothesis was considered that the mitochondrial phosphorylating enzyme is a nucleoside phosphotransferase rather than a dT kinase. Purified mitochondrial extracts were therefore incubated with several deoxyribo- and ribonucleoside 5'-monophosphates, diphosphates, and triphosphates. Either dT or dU was used as nucleoside acceptor. For control purposes, purified cytosol extracts were also incubated with various phosphate donors and nucleoside acceptors. The results of these experiments demonstrated that nucleoside 5'-monophosphates and diphosphates are not phosphate donors for either the

117

mitochondrial or cytosol phosphorylating enzymes. Both enzymes are inhibited by dTTP. Furthermore, Urd, Cyd, and Ade do not competetively inhibit the phosphorylation of ^{3}H-dU, as would be expected if these nucleosides were alternative nucleoside acceptors (85, 92). These experiments demonstrate that the mitochondrial and cytosol enzymes are dT kinases and not nucleoside phosphotransferases.

The preceding phosphorylation experiments were carried out at pH's varying from 5.5 to 9.0. The optimum pH for the cytosol dT kinase was about 8.0, whereas that for the mito-chondrial dT kinase was about 8.5. Also, the shape of the pH-activity curves differed (85).

The mitochondrial and cytosol dT kinases also differed with respect to their responses to nucleoside 5'-triphos-phates. The cytosol dT kinase utilized only ATP and dATP efficiently as phosphate donors and, in the presence of ATP, dCTP had no significant effect on the phosphorylation re-action. In contrast, the mitochondrial dT kinase utilized UTP and CTP almost as well as ATP. GTP and dATP were about half as effective as ATP. However, dCTP, dGTP, dUTP, and dTTP could not replace ATP as phosphate donors. In the presence of ATP, dCTP partially inhibited the phosphoryla-tion of ^{3}H-dT (92). Recently, Taylor, Stafford and Jones (95) and Stafford and Jones (96) found that the "adult" form of dT kinase from human tissues utilizes nucleoside triphosphates other than ATP and dATP as phosphate donors, but "fetal" and "tumor" forms of dT kinase do not. Also, Bresnick and coworkers (49) discovered several years ago that both dCTP and dTTP inhibit dT kinase activity in adult rat liver, but dCTP has little effect upon the enzymes from embryonic and regenerating liver. Several rat hepatomas were studied and they fell into 2 classes: (a) those with a dT kinase sensitive to both dCTP and dTTP; and (b) those with a dT kinase sensitive only to dTTP. The minimal devi-ation hepatomas gave results similar to adult liver, while the Novikoff and Dunning hepatomas resembled fetal and re-generating rat liver. Since the cytosol form of dT kinase predominates in tumor, fetal, and regenerating rat liver tissues and the mitochondrial form is the major activity in adult tissues, our results are in agreement with those of Jones and collaborators (95,96) and Bresnick and coworkers (49).

Glycerol Gradient Centrifugation Experiments

To determine the sedimentation coefficients, dT kinase
extracts from cytosol and mitochondrial fractions of mouse
and human cells were analyzed by centrifugation in 10-30%
(v/v) glycerol gradients. Horse liver alcohol dehydrogenase
(ADH) was used as a reference standard. Figure 1 depicts
typical glycerol gradient centrifugation experiments with
the cytosol fraction of LM cells and the mitochondrial fraction of LM(TK⁻) cells. The cytosol dT kinase sediments at
about the same rate or slightly faster than ADH. In
contrast, the mitochondrial dT kinase sediments more slowly
than the ADH marker. This result has been obtained repeatedly with crude or purified cytosol dT kinase preparations
and with all mitochondrial dT kinases from parental or dT
kinase-deficient mouse and human cell lines (92,93).
Assuming that the enzymes are all globular proteins and
that the partial specific volumes are the same as that of
ADH, the molecular weights of the dT kinases can be estimated from the sedimentation coefficients by the method of
Martin and Ames (97). The estimated molecular weight of
cytosol dT kinase is about 83,000 to 98,000; that of mitochondrial dT kinase from parental and from mutant human
and mouse lines is about 67,000 to 77,000. The estimated
molecular weight of cytosol dT kinase is in agreement with
the value obtained by Sephadex G-200 chromatography (80,000
to 100,000) (75). Thus, the molecular weight of cytosol dT
kinase appears to be slightly greater than that of the
mitochondrial enzyme.

Disc PAGE Analyses of Cytosol and Mitochondrial dT Kinase
Activities

The disc polyacrylamide gel electrophoresis (disc PAGE)
patterns of cytosol and mitochondrial dT kinases are
distinctive (Fig. 2-4). The cytosol dT kinase from parental mKS-A and LM mouse cell lines exhibits a single disc
PAGE peak with a mobility relative to the tracking-dye (Rm)
of about 0.25-0.33 (Fig. 2a, 3a). The cytosol enzyme utilizes ATP, but not CTP, GTP, or UTP as a phosphate donor in
the dT kinase reaction. Cytosol dT kinase activity is not
detected in extracts from mutant LM(TK⁻) (Fig. 3c) or mKS
(BU100) cells (not shown). In contrast, the mitochondrial
dT kinase of mutant LM(TK⁻) and mKS(BU100) cells exhibits

119

an Rm of about 0.7–0.8. This rapidly migrating mitochondrial dT kinase utilizes not only ATP, but also UTP, CTP, and GTP as phosphate donors (Fig. 3d, Fig. 4).

As expected, the mitochondrial fraction of parental mKS-A and LM mouse cells contains the 0.7–0.8 Rm activity which utilizes ATP, GTP, CTP, and UTP as phosphate donors (Fig. 2b, 3b). In addition, a second minor dT kinase activity is detected with an Rm of about 0.4. The 0.4 Rm dT kinase utilizes only ATP as phosphate donor.

The disc PAGE patterns of cytosol and mitochondrial fractions of human cells resemble those of mouse cells, with the exceptions to be described below. A single disc PAGE dT kinase peak with an Rm of 0.2–0.3 is detected in the cytosol fraction of dT kinase-positive HeLa S3 cells (Fig. 5b). This molecular form of dT kinase is also detected in the cytosol fraction of Burkitt's lymphoma, SV40-transformed human skin (W98 VaD), SV40-transformed human lung (W138 Val3A), and xeroderma pigmentosa cells (92). The single slowly migrating disc PAGE peak is observed whether disc PAGE analyses are carried out at pH 8.6, as in the experiment of Fig. 5b, or at pH 8.3 or 9.0 (not shown). The 0.2–0.3 Rm peak is also found in cytosol extracts of dT kinase-deficient HeLa(BU25) cells, but in the latter cells, the 0.2–0.3 Rm activity is barely detectable because of the very low cytosol enzyme levels in HeLa(BU25) cells (Table 4). The 0.2–0.3 Rm cytosol enzyme utilizes ATP, but not UTP as phosphate donor (Fig. 5b).

Mitochondrial extracts of HeLa(BU25) cells contain 2 dT kinase molecular species detectable by disc PAGE analysis. The faster migrating peak has an Rm of about 0.6–0.7 and utilizes ATP, UTP (Fig. 5d) or GTP (not shown) as phosphate donors. The second peak has an Rm of about 0.4 and utilizes only ATP as phosphate donor.

The mitochondrial fraction of parental HeLa S3 cells contains 3 molecular forms of dT kinase (Fig. 5a, 5c). The 2 faster migrating forms are similar in Rm to the 2 molecular forms found in the mitochondrial fraction of HeLa(BU25) cells (Fig. 5d). The third molecular form (Rm of about 0.24) resembles the cytosol enzyme, and is also present in mito-chondrial fractions of all dT kinase-positive human cell lines tested.

The proportion of total mitochondrial dT kinase activity found in the 0.24 Rm peak varies with the growth state of the cells and is relatively high when a very high specific activity enzyme is present in the cytosol fraction. This

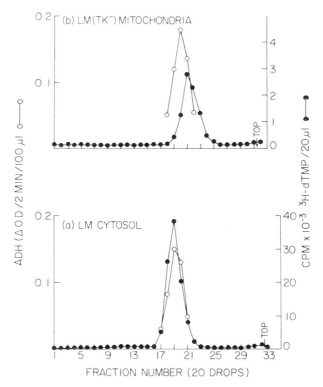

Fig. 1. *Centrifugation in 10 to 30% (v/v) glycerol
gradients of dT kinase from (a) LM cytosol (1160 µg protein)
and (b) LM(TK-) mitochondrial (1380 µg protein) fractions.*
Each tube contained 11 ml of 10-30% (v/v) glycerol in 0.15M
KCl, 10 mM 2-mercaptoethanol, 0.2 mM dT, 1.25 mM MgCl$_2$, 2.5
mM ATP, and 0.05M Tris-HCl, pH 8.0 at 25°. Five tenths ml
of dT kinase solution was layered over the glycerol and the
tubes were centrifuged for 18-20 hr. at 4° at 200,000 x g.
Horse liver alcohol dehydrogenase (ADH) (S = 5.1, M.W. =
83,000) was added to the enzyme solution as a reference
marker. Twenty drop fractions were collected from the
bottom of the centrifuge tubes into vials chilled at 0° and
portions were assayed for dT kinase activity and for ADH
(92,93). For the assay of dT kinase activity, LM cytosol
fractions were incubated 1 hr. at 38° and LM(TK-) mitochondrial fractions for 2 hr. at 38°. About 63% of the
original cytosol activity and 105% of the original mitochondrial activity were recovered from the gradients.

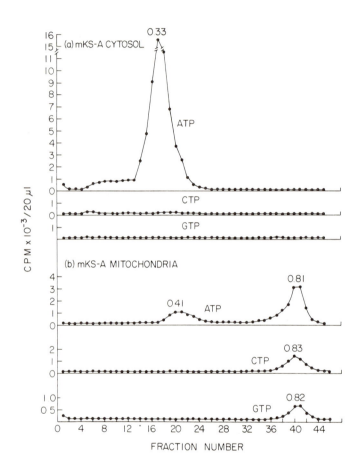

Fig. 2. *disc PAGE analyses of dT kinase activities of (a) mKS-A cytosol and (b) mKS-A mitochondrial fractions.*
Analyses were performed in 5% (w/v) N,N'-methylene bisacrylamide gels as previously described (92,93). The upper and lower buffer chambers contained 25 mM Tris-HCl, 0.192M glycine, 1 mM $MgCl_2$, 0.2 mM dT, and 10 mM 2-mercaptoethanol, at a final pH of 8.6 (at 25°). The upper buffer also contained 2.5 mM ATP, GTP, or CTP. Fifty microliters of enzyme sample was mixed with 5 µl of a sucrose-bromophenol blue solution [50% sucrose, 0.1% bromophenol blue (w/v), 1mM $MgCl_2$], the mixture was layered on top of the gels and the samples were electrophoresed at 3 ma/gel for approximately 75 min. at 4°.

At the end of the disc PAGE run, the gels were sliced in a cold room with a razor blade into 1 mm sections and the slices were immediately incubated with shaking for 1 hr. (cytosol fraction) or 2 hr. (mitochondrial fraction) at 38° in small vials containing 150 µl of dT kinase reaction mixture. When CTP or GTP were used in the upper buffer solution, CTP and GTP, respectively, were also substituted for ATP as phosphate donors in the dT kinase reaction mixture. The reaction was terminated by the addition of 25 µl of 50% trichloroacetic acid (w/v) and 20 µl aliquots were chromatographed on Whatman DE-81 paper to separate the nucleoside acceptor, ^{3}H-dT, from the product, ^{3}H-dTMP. The amount of ^{3}H-dTMP formed was determined using a Packard Tri-Carb liquid scintillation spectrometer.

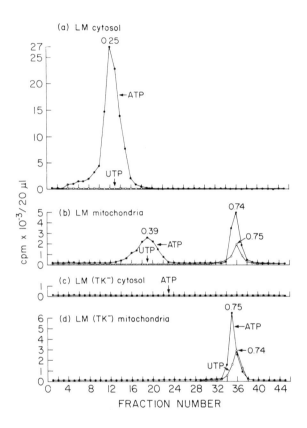

Fig. 3. *disc PAGE analyses of dT kinase activities of (a) LM cytosol; (b) LM mitochondrial; (c) LM(TK⁻) cytosol; and (d) LM(TK⁻) mitochondrial fractions.* See text and legend to Fig. 2 for experimental details.

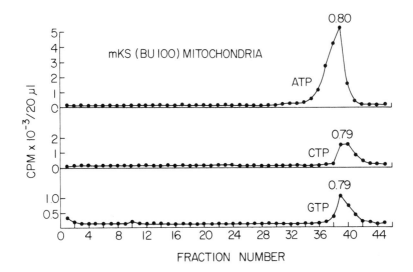

Fig. 4. *disc PAGE analysis of dT kinase activity of mKS (BU100) mitochondrial fraction.* See legend to Fig. 2 for details. ATP, CTP, or GTP were added to the upper buffer solution, and the same nucleoside triphosphate used in the upper buffer solution was employed as phosphate donor in the dT kinase reaction mixture.

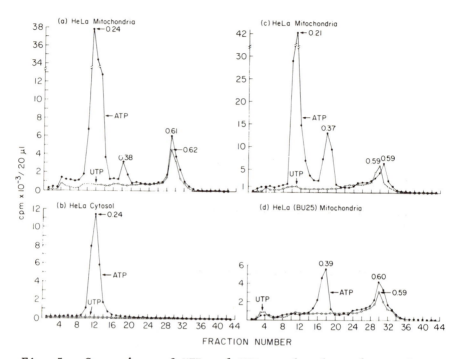

Fig. 5. *Comparison of UTP and ATP as phosphate donors for dT kinase after disc PAGE analyses of (a) purified HeLa S3 mitochondrial enzyme; (b) purified HeLa S3 cytosol enzyme; (c) crude HeLa S3 mitochondrial extract; and (d) crude HeLa(BU25) mitochondrial extract.* The mitochondrial and cytosol enzymes [(a) and (b)] were purified by 2 ammonium sulfate precipitations and extensively dialyzed against enzyme buffer containing 0.2 mM dT and 0.05M epsilon amino-caproic acid (EACA) prior to disc PAGE analysis. Enzymes analyzed in (c) and (d) are from high speed supernatant fractions of mitochondrial extracts. With each enzyme, one gel was run with 2.5 mM ATP in the upper buffer and the second gel with 2.5 mM UTP in the upper buffer. At the conclusion of the disc PAGE run, the gels were sliced and each slice was incubated at 38° with the dT kinase reaction mixture. The cytosol enzyme (b) was incubated for 1 hr. and the mitochondrial enzymes (a,c,d) for 2 hr. UTP was substituted for ATP in the dT kinase reaction mixture of the samples in which UTP was used in the upper buffer of the disc PAGE run.

molecular form of dT kinase efficiently utilizes only ATP
as phosphate donor. A portion of this 0.24 Rm mitochondrial
dT kinase of HeLa S3 cells probably results from contamination by the predominant cytosol enzyme. Evidence has been
obtained, however, indicating that contamination alone does
not account for all the 0.24 Rm activity and that this molecular form may be intrinsic to the mitochondria of dT kinase-
positive human cells (98).

It was of interest to learn whether the two dT kinase
molecular forms from HeLa(BU25) mitochondria differ in sedimentation coefficient. Therefore, HeLa(BU25) mitochondrial
extracts were centrifuged in a linear 10-30% (v/v) glycerol
gradient (Fig. 6, insert). Fractions collected from the
leading front (A,B), the center (C,D), and the light end
(E,F) of the dT kinase peak were collected and analyzed by
disc PAGE. Fig. 6 shows that the 0.4 Rm peak is predominant
in the fraction (A) from the heavy end of the glycerol
gradient and that the 0.6-0.7 Rm peak is the major activity
in fractions C-E of the gradient. Fraction F from the
light end of the gradient peak consists almost entirely of
the 0.6-0.7 Rm molecular form. From analysis of the glycerol gradient and disc PAGE experiments, it can be estimated that the 0.4 Rm and 0.6-0.7 Rm activities have sedimentation coefficients of about 5.3S (88,000 M.W.) and
4.4S (67,000 M.W.), respectively. Thus, the 0.4 Rm molecular form seems to be slightly larger than the 0.7-0.8 Rm
molecular form.

Similar experiments have been carried out with the
HeLa S3 mitochondrial dT kinase. In this instance, the
enzyme was purified by 2 ammonium sulfate precipitations
prior to glycerol gradient centrifugation (92). Several
fractions were collected from the leading front, the center,
and the light end of the dT kinase peak and analyzed by
disc PAGE. The 0.2-0.3 Rm activity was predominant in the
fraction from the heavy side; the 0.6-0.7 Rm activity was
predominant in the fraction from the center; and essentially
all of the activity in the fraction from the light side of
the glycerol gradient peak was detected in the 0.6-0.7 Rm
molecular form. The sedimentation coefficients of these
fractions were estimated to be 5.5S, 4.7S, and 4.1S, respectively. These results indicate that the 0.2-0.3 Rm
mitochondrial dT kinase activity of HeLa S3 has about the
same sedimentation coefficient as the 0.2-0.3 Rm cytosol
enzyme and is larger than the 0.6-0.7 Rm enzyme.

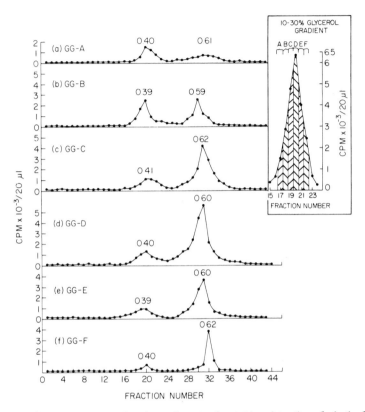

Fig. 6. *disc PAGE analysis of HeLa(BU25) mitochondrial dT kinase.* The enzyme was first centrifuged in a linear 10-30% (v/v) glycerol gradient (see legend tó Fig. 1). Fractions A to F obtained after glycerol gradient centrifugation (insert) were then analyzed by disc PAGE. Gel slices were assayed for dT kinase activity for 2 hr. at 38°. Portions of the fractions from the glycerol gradients were assayed for 1 hr. The estimated sedimentation coefficients of glycerol gradient fractions B and D were 5.3S and 4.4S, respectively, relative to an ADH marker (5.1S; M.W. = 83,000).

128

Gel Electrofocusing Experiments

Taking into account the results of the glycerol gradient centrifugation and disc PAGE analyses, it may be inferred that the 0.6-0.7 Rm mitochondrial dT kinase differs in net charge from the cytosol enzyme and from the slower migrating mitochondrial molecular forms. Gel electrofocusing experiments have been carried out to investigate this possibility. The results of preliminary experiments indicate that the HeLa S3 cytosol enzyme has a pI of about 9, the 0.6-0.7 Rm mitochondrial dT kinase has a pI of about 6, and that the 0.4 Rm activity has a pI of about 8.5. These results confirm the hypothesis that the 0.6-0.7 Rm mitochondrial dT kinase is more negatively charged under the conditions of disc PAGE than the 0.2-0.3 and the 0.4 Rm molecular forms.

Localization of dT Kinase in Mitochondria

In order to ascertain the localization of dT kinase, the mitochondria from HeLa(BU25) and HeLa S3 cells were purified and fractionated by the digitonin-lubrol method of Schnaitman and Greenawalt (99). In the case of HeLa (BU25) mitochondria, 23.8%, 74.6%, 1.5%, and 0.1% of the total dT kinase activity was recovered in the inner membrane, matrix, outer membrane, and intermembrane fractions, respectively. The specific activity of the matrix fraction was about 4-5-times greater than that of the inner membrane fraction and 30-times greater than that of the outer membrane fraction. The specific activity of the intermembrane fraction was the lowest of the fractions. Most of the activity in the matrix fraction exhibited a disc PAGE Rm of 0.7. The 0.4 Rm activity was detected in each of the mitochondrial fractions, but was most abundant in the inner membrane fraction. The HeLa S3 mitochondria contained more dT kinase activity in the outer membrane fraction, than did the HeLa (BU25) mitochondria. About 17.9%, 55.7%, 24.4%, and 2.0% of the total dT kinase activity was recovered in the inner membrane, matrix, outer membrane and intermembrane fractions, respectively. The specific activity of the matrix dT kinase was about twice as great as that of the outer membrane and inner membrane dT kinase fractions and 3 times greater than that of the intermembrane fraction. The matrix fraction contained all three mitochondrial activities. The major activity in the intermembrane and outer membrane fractions

was the 0.2-0.3 Rm activity; the major activity in the inner
membrane fraction was the 0.4 Rm enzyme. The results demonstrate that the dT kinase activities of mitochondria are
primarily associated with the inner membrane and matrix fractions and are not due merely to adsorption of cytosol enzymes
to the outer mitochondrial membrane.

Relationship of disc PAGE Peaks

It seems probable that the 0.2-0.3 Rm mitochondrial dT
kinase originates from association of the cytosol dT kinase
with mitochondrial structures. The 0.2-0.3 Rm dT kinase is
detected in mitochondria of dT kinase-positive human cells,
but not in mitochondria of mutant HeLa(BU25) cells. In
contrast, the rapidly migrating mitochondrial dT kinase
(0.6-0.7 Rm in human cells and 0.7-0.8 Rm in mouse cells)
may be a genetically distinct isozyme. This molecular form
of dT kinase differs from the cytosol enzyme in disc PAGE
mobility, sedimentation coefficient, pH-activity curve,
phosphate donor specificity, sensitivity to dCTP inhibition
and pI. The strongest evidence favoring the hypothesis
that it is a distinctive isozyme is the finding that the
rapidly migrating (0.7 Rm) dT kinase persists in the mitochondria of mKS(BU100), LM(TK⁻) and HeLa(BU25) cells, despite the loss of the principal cytosol enzyme from the
mutant cells.
The origin of the 0.4 Rm mitochondrial activity is unclear. The 0.4 Rm activity resembles the cytosol dT kinase
in sedimentation coefficient and it efficiently utilizes ATP,
but not other ribonucleoside triphosphates as phosphate
donors. The 0.4 Rm activity is present in HeLa(BU25) mitochondria, which exhibit a minor residual cytosol activity
(Rm of about 0.2), but not in the mitochondria of the two dT
kinase-deficient mouse lines, which do not contain any
detectable cytosol enzyme. Furthermore, a minor 0.4 Rm dT
kinase molecular form is present in the mitochondria of
parental, dT kinase-positive mouse lines. The 0.4 Rm molecular form could be another isozyme or a cytosol enzyme
that has been modified by the mitochondria.
Several subclones of HeLa(BU25) cells have recently
been isolated in an effort to obtain a clonal line completely
devoid of cytosol enzyme. disc PAGE analyses of these sub-
lines may enable us to confirm whether the 0.4 Rm activity
is indeed derived from the cytosol enzyme. If this is in
fact the case, it would be predicted that the 0.4 Rm activity

will not be found in those clonal lines which are totally
lacking in the cytosol dT kinase.

Site of Synthesis of the Rapidly Migrating Mitochondrial
dT Kinase

The site of synthesis of the rapidly migrating (0.6-0.7
Rm) mitochondrial dT kinase has been investigated by growing HeLa(BU25) and CV-1 (monkey kidney) cultures in media
containing ethidium bromide (EtBr). Low concentrations of
EtBr inhibit mitochondrial DNA, RNA, and protein synthesis
without inhibiting cell growth, nuclear DNA synthesis, or
nuclear DNA-dependent RNA synthesis.

Cultures of African green monkey kidney (CV-1) cells
were treated 2 days after seeding with 0.1 µg/ml EtBr. This
concentration of EtBr prevented mitochondrial DNA synthesis.
At 2 and 5 days after EtBr treatment, cultures were harvested,
fractionated into cytosol and mitochondrial fractions, and
assayed for dT kinase activity. Table 5 shows that both
control and EtBr-treated cultures grew in 7 days from 10^6
to about 13.5 x 10^6 cells. In both control and treated
cultures between the fourth and seventh days after seeding,
the cell number per culture tripled, the total cytosol dT
kinase activity per culture doubled, but the total mitochondrial dT kinase activity per culture increased 6 to 8-
fold. Also, EtBr treatment did not reduce cytosol and mitochondrial dT kinase specific activities, expressed as enzyme units per 10^6 cells or per µg protein.

Similar experiments were carried out with HeLa(BU25)
cells (Table 6). Two days after seeding 10^6 cells, cultures
were treated with 0.15 or 0.30 µg/ml EtBr. Cultures were
harvested 7 days after seeding. The control and EtBr-treated
cultures grew to 15.7 x 10^6 cells and about 11 x 10^6 cells
per culture, respectively, in 7 days. Nevertheless, the
total mitochondrial dT kinase activity and the mitochondrial
dT kinase specific activity of EtBr-treated cultures exceeded
those of control cultures. These results suggest that the
mitochondrial-specific dT kinase is coded by nuclear genes
and translated on cytoplasmic polyribosomes. Thus, the
mitochondrial dT kinase resembles other isozymes (*e.g.*, RNA
polymerase, DNA polymerase, malate dehydrogenase, cytochrome
c, and aminopeptidase) which are localized in mitochondria
but synthesized on polyribosomes and coded by nuclear genes
(100-105).

131

TABLE 5

Effect of Ethidium Bromide (EtBr) on the Cytosol and Mitochondrial
dT Kinase Activities of CV-1 Cells[a]

Cells/Culture and dT Kinase Activity	4 Days after Seeding		7 Days after Seeding	
	Control	EtBr	Control	EtBr
Cells/Culture (10^6)	4.9	4.4	13.2	13.8
Cytosol activity per 10^6 cells	570	930	510	490
Mitochondrial activity per 10^6 cells	29.6	22.2	61.7	61.7
Cytosol activity per μg protein	5.1	5.4	7.4	11.0
Mitochondrial activity per μg protein	1.1	1.0	3.8	4.0
Total cytosol activity per culture	2,800	4,100	6,700	6,800
Total mitochondrial activity per culture	140	100	820	860

[a] Cells were seeded at 10^6 cells/culture. Two days after seeding, when the cell number per culture was 1.6 x 10^6, 0.1 μg/ml EtBr was added to experimental cultures. dT kinase activity was expressed as picomoles dUMP formed in 15 min. at 38°.

TABLE 6

Effect of Ethidium Bromide (EtBr) Treatment for 5 Days on the Cytosol and Mitochondrial dT Kinase Activities of HeLa(BU25) Cells[a]

Cells per Culture and dT Kinase Activity	Control	EtBr-Treated 0.15 µg/ml	0.30 µg/ml
Cells (10^6) per culture	15.7	10.3	11.6
Cytosol activity per 10^6 cells	6.9	9.9	8.8
Mitochondrial activity per 10^6 cells	30.9	56.4	58.3
Cytosol activity per µg protein	0.1	0.2	0.2
Mitochondrial activity per µg protein	3.0	5.4	5.2
Total cytosol activity per culture	110	100	100
Total mitochondrial activity per culture	490	590	680

[a] 0.9×10^6 cells were seeded per culture. Two days later, when the cultures contained 1.2×10^6 cells, the media were changed and EtBr added to experimental cultures. On days 5 and 6 after seeding, control cultures contained 5.2 and 15.0 x 10^6 cells/culture; cultures treated with 0.15 µg/ml EtBr contained 6.9 and 10.5 x 10^6 cells/culture; and cultures treated with 0.30 µg/ml EtBr contained 6.0 and 10.3 x 10^6 cells/culture. Cells were harvested 7 days after seeding and extracts prepared for dT kinase assays. Activity expressed as picomoles dUMP formed in 30 min. at 38°.

A 0.7 Rm dT kinase activity has not been detected in
the cytosol fraction of any cell line so far tested. Nor
has the 0.7 Rm activity been found in detergent-treated
microsome fractions of HeLa S3 or HeLa(BU25) cells. This
unexpected result suggests that the mitochondrial-specific
0.7 Rm dT kinase exists only transiently and at a very low
concentrations in the cytosol fraction before being trans-
ported to and packaged in mitochondria.

Cellular Localization of dT Kinases Induced During Liver
Regeneration, After Hormonal Stimulation, and After Virus
Infection

The mitochondrial dT kinase is the principal cellular
enzyme in adult liver. When DNA synthesis and tissue growth
are stimulated by partial hepatectomy, the activity of the
mitochondrial enzyme per gram of liver remains constant,
but the activity of the cytosol enzyme increases about 40-
fold (42,106). Also, it is the cytosol and not the mitochondrial enzyme which exhibits a high turnover rate.
Adelstein, Baldwin, and Kohn (106) found after injection of
puromycin into 10-day-old mice that the cytosol dT kinase
activity of liver decreased with an apparent half-life of
one day, but the mitochondrial dT kinase activity decreased
very slowly.

ACTH administration to guinea pigs also induces the
rapid synthesis of the cytosol, but not the mitochondrial
dT kinase (107). Preliminary experiments have been carried
out in our laboratory on virus-infected cells. These
experiments indicate that the dT kinase induced after SV40
infection is mostly the cytosol enzyme. Also, the dT kinases
with distinctive disc PAGE mobilities that are induced after
vaccinia and herpes simplex infections are mainly localized
in the cytosol cell fraction (Jorgensen, G.J. and Kit, S.,
unpublished experiments).

Stafford and coworkers (95,96) have observed that the
cytosol dT kinase accounts for the high enzyme levels in
fetal and neoplastic tissues. Indeed, they have suggested
that the cytosol dT kinase may be equated with the "fetal"
molecular form of this enzyme and that the mitochondrial
dT kinase corresponds to the "adult" molecular form.

A variety of fetal antigens have been described in
human tumors and it has been shown that certain fetal
antigens are derepressed in cells undergoing carcinogenic

transformation. The observations that fetal antigens are re-expressed in tumors has both practical and theoretical implications. Unfortunately, however, biological functions have not been assigned to the derepressed fetal antigens. Hence, their roles in promoting neoplastic growth are unclear. Increased dT kinase activity is associated with the initiation of DNA synthesis. Thus, in contrast to the expression of fetal antigens, the expression of the fetal (cytosol) form of dT kinase can be rationalized in relation to growth and neoplasia.

Significance of Mitochondrial dT Kinase

Experiments with dT kinase-deficient cells demonstrate that a distinctive organelle-specific molecular form of dT kinase exists in mitochondria. In addition, the experiments with dT kinase-positive cell lines indicate that a cytosol-like enzyme and, possibly, a modified dT kinase, may be packaged by mitochondria. The mitochondrial dT kinases could contribute to mitochondrial autonomy. The mitochondrial-specific dT kinases also provide an interesting marker for studies on mitochondrial biogenesis and nuclear-cytoplasmic relationships.

It is thought that mitochondrial DNA synthesis takes place late in the S-phase or in the G-2 phase of the cell cycle (108,109). Mitochondrial proteins coded by nuclear genes and synthesized on polyribosomes are probably made prior to the synthesis of mitochondrial DNA. In contrast, proteins translated on mitoribosomes from mitochondrial DNA are made after mitochondrial DNA is synthesized. The latter proteins consist of inner membrane proteins and, possibly, a mitochondrial repressor of the nuclear genes that specify mitochondrial enzymes (100,103,104).

Mitochondrial DNA and protein synthesis can be selectively inhibited by EtBr and chloramphenicol, respectively. Treatment of cells with these drugs prevents inner membrane protein and mitochondrial repressor synthesis. As a result, an enhanced synthesis of derepressed nuclear-coded mitochondrial proteins can be observed. For example, after specific inhibition of mitochondrial protein synthesis in yeast and Neurospora, respectively, ATPase and RNA polymerase accumulate in the post-ribosomal supernatant fraction (100,104). In our experiments with EtBr-treated CV-1 and HeLa(BU25) cells, mitochondrial DNA synthesis (and presumably protein formation) were inhibited for about 4 cellular replication cycles. The synthesis and packaging of mitochondrial dT kinase continued during this time. In drug-treated HeLa (BU25) cells, mitochondrial dT kinase synthesis was enhanced, suggesting derepression (Table 6). It would be interesting to learn whether longer treatments with EtBr would ultimately lead to a deficiency in inner membrane proteins and an accumulation of the presumptive mitochondrial dT kinase in the cytosol fraction.

Another consequence of disturbed mitochondrial DNA and protein synthesis is the derepression of nuclear genes coding for glycolytic enzymes (110). This suggests that the expression of genes controlling anaerobic energy production may also be regulated by a mitochondrial repressor. Koobs (110) has speculated that proteins functioning in "mitosis" may be under similar control. If the cytosol dT kinase and "fetal" antigens are among the "mitotic" proteins, then inactivation of the mitochondrial repressor could account for some of the characteristic metabolic changes associated with neoplasia.

Regardless of the merits of the preceding speculations, it is apparent that more information is needed on the control of the synthesis of cytosol and mitochondrial dT kinases. Elucidation of these control mechanisms would advance our understanding of normal and abnormal growth.

Presented by Saul Kit. This investigation was aided by Grants Q-163 and Q-475 from the Robert A. Welch Foundation and by USPHS Grants CA-06656-11, CA-10893 and 1-k6-AI-2352 from the National Cancer Institute and the National Institute of Allergy and Infectious Diseases.

References

1. Kessel, D. and I. Wodinsky. Thymidine kinase as a determinant of the response to 5-fluoro-2'-deoxyuridine in transplantable murine leukemias. Mol. Pharm. 6: 251 (1970).
2. Kaufman, H.E. and C. Heidelberger. Therapeutic antiviral action of 5-trifluoromethyl-2'-deoxyuridine in herpes simplex keratitis. Science 145: 585 (1964).

3. Freese, E. The specific mutagenic effect of base analogues on Phage T4. J. Mol. Biol. 1: 87 (1959).
4. Eisenberg, R.J. and A.B. Pardee. Gene photoinactivation in *Escherichia coli* which contain 5-bromodeoxyuridine-substituted DNA. Biochim. Biophys. Acta 204: 112 (1970).
5. Kit, S. and T.C. Hsu. Relative stability to thermal denaturation of deoxyribonucleic acid (DNA) preparations containing bromodeoxyuridine. Biochem. Biophys. Res. Commun. 5: 120 (1961).
6. Baldwin, R.L. and E.M. Shooter. The alkaline transition of BU-containing DNA and its bearing on the replication of DNA. J. Mol. Biol. 7: 511 (1963).
7. Puck, T.T. and F.-T. Kao. Genetics of somatic mammalian cells. V. Treatment with 5-bromodeoxyuridine and visible light for isolation of nutritionally deficient mutants. Proc. Nat. Acad. Sci. USA 58: 1227 (1967).
8. Boettiger, D. and H.M. Temin. Light inactivation of focus formation by chick embryo fibroblasts infected with avian sarcoma virus in the presence of bromodeoxyuridine. Nature 228: 622 (1970).
9. Simon, E.H. Transfer of DNA from parent to progeny in a tissue culture line of human carcinoma of the cervix (strain HeLa). J. Mol. Biol. 3: 101 (1961).
10. Cleaver, J.E. and R.B. Painter. Evidence for repair replication of HeLa cell DNA damaged by ultraviolet light. Biochem. Biophys. Acta 161: 552 (1968).
11. Lark, K.G. Regulation of chromosome replication and segregation in bacteria. Bact. Rev. 30: 3 (1966).
12. O'Sullivan, A. and N. Sueoka. Sequential replication of the *Bacillus subtilis* chromosome. IV. Genetic mapping by density transfer experiment. J. Mol. Biol. 27: 349 (1967).
13. McKenna, W.G. and M. Masters. Biochemical evidence for the bidirectional replication of DNA in *Escherichia coli*. Nature 240: 536 (1972).
14. Price, K.E., R.E. Buck and J. Lein. Incidence of antineoplastic activity among antibiotics found to be inducers of lysogenic bacteria. Antimicrobiol. Agents Chemother. 4: 505 (1964).
15. Rothschild, H. and P.H. Black. Analysis of SV40-induced transformation of hamster kidney tissue *in vitro*. VII. Induction of SV 40 virus from transformed hamster cell clones by various agents. Virol. 42: 251 (1970).

16. Teich, N., D.R. Lowry, J.W. Hartley and W.P. Rowe. Studies of the mechanism of induction of infectious murine leukemia virus from AKR mouse embryo cell lines by 5-iododeoxyuridine and 5-bromodeoxyuridine. Virol. 51: 163 (1973).

17. Aaronson, S.A., G.J. Todaro, E.M. Scolnick. Induction of murine C-type viruses from clonal lines of virus-free BALB/3T3 cells. Science 174: 157 (1971).

18. Aaronson, S.A. Chemical induction of focus-forming virus from nonproducer cells transformed by murine sarcoma virus. Proc. Nat. Acad. Sci. USA 68: 3069 (1971).

19. Klement, V., M.O. Nicolson and R.J. Huebner. Rescue of the genome of focus-forming virus from rat nonproductive lines by 5-bromodeoxyuridine. Nature 234: 12 (1971).

20. Silagi, S., D. Beju, J. Wrathall and E. DeHarven. Tumorigenicity, immunogenicity, and virus production in mouse melanoma cells treated with 5-bromodeoxyuridine. Proc. Nat. Acad. Sci. USA 69: 3443 (1972).

21. Stewart, S.E., G. Kasnic, Jr., C. Draycott and T. Ben. Activation of virus in human tumors by 5-iododeoxyuridine and dimethylsulfoxide. Science 175: 198 (1972).

22. Gerber, P. Activation of Epstein-Barr virus by 5-bromodeoxyuridine in "virus-free" human cells. Proc. Nat. Acad. Sci. USA 69: 83 (1972).

23. Hamper, B., J.G. Derge, L.M. Martos and J.L. Walker. Synthesis of Epstein-Barr virus after activation of the viral genome in a "virus-negative" human lymphoblastoid cell (Raji) made resistant to 5-bromodeoxyuridine. Proc. Nat. Acad. Sci. USA 69: 78 (1972).

24. Stockdale, F., K. Okazaki, M. Nameroff and H. Holtzer. 5-bromodeoxyuridine: Effect on myogenesis *in vitro*. Science 146: 533 (1964).

25. Abbott, J. and H. Holtzer. The loss of phenotypic traits by differentiated cells. V. The effect of 5-bromodeoxyuridine on cloned chondrocytes. Proc. Nat. Acad. Sci. USA 59: 1144 (1968).

26. Holthausen, H.S., S. Chacko, E.A. Davidson and H. Holtzer. Effect of 5-bromodeoxyuridine on expression of cultured chondrocytes grown *in vitro*. Proc. Nat. Acad. Sci. USA 63: 864 (1969).

27. Bischoff, R. and H. Holtzer. Inhibition of hyaluronic acid synthesis by BUDR in culture of chick ammion cells. Anat. Rec. 160: 317 (1968).

28. Coleman, A.W., D. Kunkel, I. Werner and J.R. Coleman. Cellular differentiation *in vitro*. Perturbation by halogenated deoxyribonucleosides. J. Cell. Biol. 39: 27a (1968).
29. Koyama, H. and T. Ono. Effect of 5-bromodeoxyuridine on hyaluronic acid synthesis of a clonal hybrid line of mouse and Chinese hamster in culture. J. Cell. Physiol. 78: 265 (1971).
30. Scher, W., H.D. Preisler and C. Friend. Hemoglobin synthesis in murine virus-induced leukemic cells *in vitro*. III. Effects of 5-bromodeoxyuridine, dimethyl-formamide, and dimethylsulfoxide. J. Cell. Physiol. 81: 63 (1973).
31. Turkington, R.W., G.C. Majumder and M. Riddle. Inhibition of mammary gland differentiation *in vitro* by 5-bromo-2'-deoxyuridine. J. Biol. Chem. 246: 1814 (1971).
32. Stellwagen, R.H. and G.M. Tomkins. Differential effect of 5-bromodeoxyuridine on the concentrations of specific enzymes in hepatoma cells in culture. Proc. Nat. Acad. Sci. USA 68: 1147 (1971).
33. Jones, T.C. and W.F. Dove. Photosensitization of transcription by bromodeoxyuridine substitution. J. Mol. Biol. 64: 409 (1972).
34. Lin, S.-Y. and A.D. Riggs. Lac operator analogues: Bromodeoxyuridine substitution in the lac operator affects the rate of dissociation of the lac repressor. Proc. Nat. Acad. Sci. USA 69: 2574 (1972).
35. Woodland, H.R. The phosphorylation of thymidine by oocytes and eggs of *Xenopus laevis daudin*. Biochim. Biophys. Acta 186: 1 (1969).
36. Whitlock, J.P. Jr., R. Kaufman and R. Baserga. Changes in thymidine kinase and α-amylase activity during iso-proterenol-stimulated DNA synthesis in mouse salivary gland. Cancer Res. 28: 2211 (1968).
37. Thomson, M.J., M.R. Garland and J.F. Richards. Hormonal effects on thymidine kinase activity of estrogen-dependent tumors in the rat. Cancer Res. 33: 220 (1973).
38. Garland, M.R., T. Ng and J.F. Richards. Hormonal effects on thymidine kinase activity in normal rat adrenal and in hormone-dependent adrenal carcinomas. Cancer Res. 31: 1348 (1971).
39. Masui, H. and L.D. Garen. On the mechanism of action of adrenocorticotrophic hormone. Stimulation of deoxyribonucleic acid polymerase and thymidine kinase activities in adrenal glands. J. Biol. Chem. 245: 2627 (1970).

40. Epstein, S., C. Esanu and M.S. Raben. The effect of growth hormone and cortisone on thymidine kinase activity in rat adipose tissue. Biochim. Biophys. Acta 186: 280 (1969).

41. Brookes, V.J. and C.M. Williams. Thymidine kinase and thymidylate kinase in relation to the endocrine control of insect diapause and development. Proc. Nat. Acad. Sci. USA 53: 770 (1965).

42. Baugnet-Mahieu, L., R. Goutier and M. Semal. Studies on the intracellular distribution of thymidine phosphorylating kinase activities in regenerating rat liver. Europ. J. Biochem. 4: 323 (1968).

43. Bresnick, E., K.D. Mainigi, R. Buccino and S.S. Burleson. Studies on deoxythymidine kinase of regenerating rat liver and *Escherichia coli*. Cancer Res. 30: 2502 (1970).

44. Cihak, A., H. Vesela and F. Sorm. Thymidine kinase and polyribosome distribution in regenerating rat liver following 5-azacytidine. Biochim. Biophys. Acta 166: 277 (1968).

45. Bresnick, E., S.S. Williams and H. Mosse. Rates of turnover of deoxythymidine kinase and its template RNA in regenerating and control liver. Cancer Res. 27: 469 (1967).

46. Mayfield, E.D., Jr., R.A. Liebelt and E. Bresnick. Activities of enzymes of deoxyribonucleic acid synthesis after unilateral nephrectomy. Cancer Res. 27: 1652 (1967).

47. Machovich, R. and O. Greengard. Thymidine kinase in rat tissues during growth and differentiation. Biochim. Biophys. Acta 286: 375 (1972).

48. Klemperer, H.G. and G.R. Haynes. Thymidine kinase in rat liver during development. Biochem. J. 108: 541 (1968).

49. Bresnick, E., U.B. Thompson, H.P. Morris and A.G. Liebelt. Inhibition of thymidine kinase activity in liver and hepatomas by dTTP and dCTP. Biochem. Biophys. Res. Commun. 16: 278 (1964).

50. Sneider, T.W., V.R. Potter and H.P. Morris. Enzymes of thymidine triphosphate synthesis in selected Morris hepatomas. Cancer Res. 29: 40 (1969).

51. Gordon, H.L., T.J. Bardos, Z.F. Chmielewicz and J.L. Ambrus. Comparative study of the thymidine kinase and thymidylate kinase activities and of the feedback inhibition of thymidine kinase in normal and neoplastic human tissue. Cancer Res. 28: 2068 (1968).

52. Roberts, D. and T.C. Hall. Enzyme activities and deoxy-nucleoside utilization of leukemic leukocytes in relation to drug therapy and resistance. Cancer Res. 29: 166 (1969).

53. Weinstock, I.M. and M.Y. Dju. Thymidine phosphorylation and thymidylate kinase in developing breast muscle of normal and dystrophic chickens. Biochim. Biophys. Acta 232: 5 (1971).

54. Tanooka, H., H. Terano and H. Otsuka. Increase in thymidine, thymidylate and deoxycytidine kinase activities during germination of bacterial spores. Biochim. Biophys. Acta 228: 26 (1971).

55. Hildebrandt, A. and H.W. Sauer. Thymidine phosphorylation in the cell cycle of *Physarum polycephalum* and the effect of 5-fluoro-2'-deoxyuridine and hydroxyurea. Biochim. Biophys. Acta 294: 8 (1973).

56. Nagano, H. and Y. Mano. Thymidine kinase, thymidylate kinase and ^{32}Pi and [^{14}C] thymidine incorporation into DNA during early embryogenesis of the sea urchin. Biochim. Biophys. Acta 157: 546 (1968).

57. Kit, S., R.A. deTorres and D.R. Dubbs. Arabinofurano-sylcytosine-induced stimulation of thymidine kinase and deoxycytidylic deaminase activities in mammalian cultures. Cancer Res. 26: 1859 (1966).

58. Stubblefield, E. and S. Murphree. Synchronized mammalian cell cultures. II. Thymidine kinase activity in colcemid synchronized fibroblasts. Exp. Cell. Res. 48: 652 (1967).

59. Sachsenmaier, W., D.V. Fournier and K.F. Gürtler. Periodic thymidine kinase production in synchronous plasmodia of *Physarum polycephalum*: Inhibition by actinomycin and actidon. Biochem. Biophys. Res. Commun. 27: 655 (1967).

60. Brent, T.P., J.A.V. Butler and A.R. Crathorn. Variations in phosphokinase activities during the cell cycle in synchronous populations of HeLa cells. Nature 207: 176 (1965).

61. Kit, S., D.R. Dubbs and P.M. Frearson. Decline of thymidine kinase activity in stationary phase mouse fibroblasts. J. Biol. Chem. 240: 2565 (1965).

62. Kit, S., D.R. Dubbs, L.J. Piekarski and T.C. Hsu. Deletion of thymidine kinase activity from L cells resistant to bromodeoxyuridine. Exp. Cell. Res. 31: 297 (1963).

63. Dubbs, D.R. and S. Kit. Effect of prolonged cultivation of SV40-transformed mouse cells in bromodeoxyuridine or pretreatment with mitomycin C on rescue of SV40. Int'l J. of Cancer 6: 223 (1970).

64. Pasztor, L.M. and F. Hu. 5-Bromodeoxyuridine tolerant melanoma cells in culture. Cytobios 4: 145 (1971).

65. Davidson, R.L. and M.D. Bick. Bromodeoxyuridine dependence--a new mutation in mammalian cells. Proc. Nat. Acad. Sci. USA 70: 138 (1973).

66. Kit, S., D.R. Dubbs and P.M. Frearson. HeLa cells resistant to bromodeoxyuridine and deficient in thymidine kinase activity. Int'l J. of Cancer 1: 19 (1966).

67. Sell, E.K. and R.S. Krooth. Tabulation of somatic cell hybrids formed between lines of cultured cells. J. Cell. Physiol. 80: 453 (1972).

68. Littlefield, J. The use of drug resistant markers to study the hybridization of mouse fibroblasts. Exp. Cell Res. 41: 190 (1966).

69. Davidson, R. and B. Ephrussi. A selective system for the isolation of hybrids between L cells and normal cells. Nature 205: 1170 (1965).

70. Migeon, B.R. and B. Childs. Hybridization of mammalian somatic cells. In: A.G. Steinberg and A.G. Bearns (Editors), Progress in Medical Genetics, Vol. VII. Grune and Stratton, Inc. New York (1970), pp. 1-24.

71. Shows, T.B. Genetics of human-mouse somatic cell hybrids: Linkage of human genes for lactate dehydrogenase-A and esterase-A$_4$. Proc. Nat. Acad. Sci. USA 69: 348 (1972).

72. Miller, O.J., P.W. Allderdice, D.A. Miller, W.R. Breg and B.R. Migeon. Human thymidine kinase gene locus: Assignment to chromosome 17 in a hybrid of man and mouse cells. Science 173: 244 (1971).

73. Green, H., R. Wang, O. Kehinde and M. Meuth. Multiple human TK chromosomes in human-mouse somatic cell hybrids. Nature New Biol. 234: 138 (1971).

74. Harris, H., O.J. Miller, G. Klein, P. Worst and T. Tachibana. Suppression of malignancy by cell fusion. Nature 233: 363 (1969).

75. Kit, S. and D.R. Dubbs. "Enzyme Induction by Viruses", S. Karger, Basel Switzerland (1969), pp. 1-114.

76. Buchan, A., D.H. Watson, D.R. Dubbs and S. Kit. Serological study of a mutant of herpes virus unable to stimulate thymidine kinase. J. Virol. 5: 817 (1970).

142

77. Thouless, M.E. Serological properties of thymidine kinase produced in cells infected with type 1 or type 2 herpes virus. J. Gen. Virol. 17: 307 (1972).
78. Buchan, A. and D.H. Watson. The immunological specificity of thymidine kinases in cells infected by viruses of the herpes group. J. Gen. Virol. 4: 461 (1969).
79. Kit, S., K. Nakajima and D.R. Dubbs. Origin of thymidine kinase in adenovirus-infected human cell lines. J. Virol. 5: 446 (1970).
80. Somers, K. and S. Kit. Enhanced DNA synthesis and enzyme activities in cells infected with murine sarcoma virus (MSV). Bact. Proc. (1970), p. 200 (abstract).
81. Munyon, W., R. Buchsbaum, E. Paoletti, J. Mann, E. Kraiselburd and D. Davis. Electrophoresis of thymidine kinase activity synthesized by cells transformed by herpes simplex virus. Virol. 49: 683 (1972).
82. Munyon, W., E. Kraiselburd, D. Davis and J. Mann. Transfer of thymidine kinase to thymidine kinaseless L cells by infection with ultraviolet irradiated herpes simplex virus. J. Virol. 7: 813 (1971).
83. Duff, R. and F. Rapp. Oncogenic transformation of hamster cells after exposure to herpes simplex virus type 2. Nature New Biol. 233: 48 (1971).
84. Rothschild, H. and P.H. Black. Effect of loss of thymidine kinase activity on the tumorigenicity of clones of SV40-transformed hamster cells. Proc. Nat. Acad. Sci. USA 67: 1042 (1970).
85. Kit, S., L.A. Kaplan, W.-C. Leung and D. Trkula. Mitochondrial thymidine kinase of bromodeoxyuridine-resistant, kinase-deficient HeLa(BU25) cells. Biochem. Biophys. Res. Commun. 49: 1561 (1972).
86. Kit, S. and Y. Minekawa. Mitochondrial thymidine-deoxyuridine-phosphorylating activity and the replication of mitochondrial DNA. Cancer Res. 32: 2277 (1972).
87. Clayton, D.A. and R.L. Teplitz. Intracellular mosaicism (nuclear-/mitochondrial[+]) for thymidine kinase in mouse L cells. J. Cell. Sci. 10: 487 (1972).
88. Attardi, B. and G. Attardi. Persistence of thymidine kinase activity in mitochondria of a thymidine kinase-deficient derivative of mouse L cells. Proc. Nat. Acad. Sci. USA 69: 2874 (1972).
89. Berk, A.J., B.J. Meyer and D.A. Clayton. Mitochondrial-specific thymidine kinase. Arch. Biochem. and Biophys. 154: 563 (1973).

90. Berk, A.J. and D.A. Clayton. A genetically distinct thymidine kinase in mammalian mitochondria. Exclusive labelling of mitochondrial deoxyribonucleic acid. J. Biol. Chem. 248: 2722 (1973).
91. Swinton, D.C. and P.C. Hanawalt. *In vivo* specific labelling of *Chlamydomonas* chloroplast DNA. J. Cell. Biol. 54: 592 (1972).
92. Kit, S., W.-C. Leung and D. Trkula. Properties of mitochondrial thymidine kinases of parental and enzyme-deficient HeLa cells. Arch. Biochem. Biophys. (in press).
93. Kit, S., W.-C. Leung and D. Trkula. Distinctive properties of mitochondrial thymidine (dT) kinase from bromodeoxyuridine (dBU)-resistant mouse lines. Biochem Biophys. Res. Commun. (in press).
94. Cohen, S.S. Are/were mitochondria and chloroplasts microorganisms? Am. Scientist 58: 281 (1970).
95. Taylor, A.T., M.A. Stafford and O.W. Jones. Properties of thymidine kinase partially purified from human fetal and adult tissue. J. Biol. Chem. 247: 1930 (1972).
96. Stafford, M.A. and O.W. Jones. The presence of "fetal" thymidine kinases in human tumors. Biochim. Biophys. Acta. 277: 439 (1972).
97. Martin, R.G. and B.N. Ames. A method for determining the sedimentation behavior of enzymes: Application to protein mixtures. J. Biol. Chem. 236: 1372 (1961).
98. Kit, S., W.-C. Leung and L.A. Kaplan. Distinctive molecular forms of thymidine kinase in mitochondria of normal and bromodeoxyuridine-resistant HeLa cells. Europ. J. Biochem. (in press).
99. Schnaitman, C. and J.W. Greenawalt. Enzymatic properties of the inner and outer membranes of rat liver mitochondria. J. Cell. Biol. 38: 158 (1968).
100. Barath, Z. and H. Küntzel. Induction of mitochondrial RNA polymerase in *Neurospora crassa*. Nature New. Biol. 240: 195 (1972).
101. Scandalios, J.G. and M.A. Campeau. Mutant aminopeptidases in Pisum. II. Nuclear gene control of a mitochondrial isozyme. Mutation Res. 14: 397 (1972).
102. Criss, W.E. A review of isozymes and cancer. Cancer Res. 31: 1523 (1971).
103. Borst, P. Mitochondrial nucleic acids. Ann. Rev. Biochem. 41: 333 (1972).

104. Tzagoloff, A., M.S. Rubin and M.F. Sierra. Biosynthesis of mitochondrial enzymes. Biochim. Biophys. Acta 301: 71 (1973).
105. Ch'ih, J.J. and G.F. Kalf. Studies in the biosynthesis of the DNA polymerase of rat liver mitochondria. Arch. Biochem. Biophys. 133: 38 (1969).
106. Adelstein, S.J., C. Baldwin and H.I. Kohn. Thymidine kinase in mouse liver: Variations in soluble and mitochondrial-associated activity that are dependent on age, regeneration, starvation, and treatment with actinomycin D and puromycin. Developmental Biology 26: 537 (1971).
107. Masui, H. and L.D. Garen. On the mechanism of action of adrenocorticotrophic hormone. The stimulation of thymidine kinase activity with altered properties and changed subcellular distribution. J. Biol. Chem. 246: 5407 (1971).
108. Bosmann, H.B. Mitochondrial biochemical events in a synchronized mammalian cell population. J. Biol. Chem. 246: 3817 (1971).
109. Koch, J. and E.L.R. Stokstad. Incorporation of [3H]-thymidine into nuclear and mitochondrial DNA in synchronized mammalian cells. Europ. J. Biochem. 3: 1 (1967).
110. Koobs, D.H. Phosphate mediation of the Crabtree and Pasteur effects. Science 178: 127 (1972).

TRANSFER RNA's AS REGULATORY MOLECULES: AN ASSESSMENT
AFTER A DECADE

Ernest Borek

Introduction

It is ten years ago almost to the day that we suggested
that modifications of tRNA's must serve some regulatory
function (1). This, then brash, suggestion was rooted in
totally unexpected observations made independently by two
of my associates. Dr. Erwin Fleissner observed that extracts
of peas can hypermethylate *in vitro* tRNA isolated from
E. Coli which had been fully methylated by the bacterial
enzymes *in vivo* (2). Dr. P.R. Srinivasan observed the same
interactions of indigenously fully methylated *E. Coli* B tRNA
with a variety of heterologous enzyme extracts (3). These
observations implied: Species specific modifications of the
tRNA's and, in turn, a species specificity of the tRNA
structures themselves.

Our suggestion for a species specific regulatory role
for the tRNA's was not in accord with the prevalent
Zeitgeist. Since the genetic code was universal, not species
specific, the tRNA's also were assumed to be universal.
Indeed, hemoglobin was claimed to have been synthesized *in
vitro* with the complement of tRNA's from *E. Coli* B (4). This
was concluded from matchings of crude peptide maps. Only
years later was it shown by more refined analyses that
hemoglobin so synthesized is replete with faulty amino acid
insertions (5).

Advance in our understanding of the relation between the
modification of tRNA structure and its function was retarded
by two factors: The first is the intrinsic complexity of the
tRNA modifying enzymes; their number is over fifty[1]. Those

---

[1]*It is interesting to contemplate the simplicity of the
synthesis of the primary sequence of tRNA, probably by a
single enzyme, against the complexity of its modification by
over two scores of enzymes. These contemporary enzymes which*

examined are highly complex in structure and in the recognition signals they require for interaction with tRNA. Moreover, many of the enzymes, especially in eukaryotes are quite unstable. Furthermore, early attempts at correlation of modification and function were essentially fruitless and discouraging. The reasons for this should have been obvious. All early work was done with mixtures of methylated and unmethylated tRNA's isolated from methionine starved *E. Coli* with relaxed control over RNA synthesis (7). Furthermore, all early probes were done with *in vitro* reactions forced to completion with a variety of artifactual manipulations. Subtlety which may be required for regulation could not be revealed by these crude attempts.

The cascade of publications from a few laboratories reporting no apparent functions for modification of tRNA discouraged investigators from sustained efforts in this area for a long time.

Regulation of Transcription

The best documented evidence for control by a specific modification of tRNA comes from the laboratory of Bruce Ames. This is appropriate since he was one of the first to suggest a regulatory role for transfer RNA on the biosynthetic operons of amino acids (8). From studies of the variety of mutants of the histidine pathway in *Salmonella typhimurium*, Ames came to the conclusion that the concentrations of charged histidyl tRNA^{his} *in vivo* regulate the transcription of the messenger RNA for the enzymes of the histidine pathway. One class of mutants, which he called hisT, was found which are continously derepressed. Analysis revealed that these mutants contain the same amount of charged tRNA^{his} as the wild type organism in which the histidine operon is inducible. This was baffling until Ames and his group discovered that the tRNA^{his} in the hisT mutant has an altered chromatographic mobility.

modify tRNA must represent the summation of long evolvement. During this evolution the enzymes became complex and some acquired synthetic finesse: Consider the complexity of the stepwise synthesis of thymine of DNA and the simplicity of the reaction for the synthesis of thymine in tRNA discovered by my student Dr. Lewis R. Mandel (6). It is a one step carbon-to-carbon methylation.

148

The observation was followed up by a heroic undertaking
of the isolation of the tRNA of the anomolous mutant and the
determination of its sequence. It appears that two uridines
in the anticodon loop are not modified to pseudouridines (Ψ)
in the mutant, differing from the tRNA^{his} in the wild type
inducible organism where these two bases are modified (9)
(Fig. 1). This is an extraordinarily significant finding
for several reasons. First of all, it serves to emphasize
that profound effects on function can accrue from such
slight modifications or lack of modification as the conversion of two out of some 80 bases. Of course, such a
modification of transfer RNA appears to be minor only in
two dimensional structure. There is mounting evidence that
recognition or interaction of tRNA's with a variety of
proteins is rooted not only in sequence but also in the
conformation of the tRNA molecules. Thus, while the change
of two uridine residues to pseudouridine appears to be
trivial, its effect on the interaction of tRNA with some
repressor protein or with DNA may be large. The second
point which became clear from the inspired and patient
work of Ames, is the absolute need for analysis of isolated,
homogeneous specific tRNA's before any conclusions on alterations of structure can be drawn. Consider how useless and
misleading it would be to analyze the total population of
tRNA's from the hisT mutant. Let us assume that there are
about an average of four Ψ residues per tRNA. If we assume
further that in *Salmonella* there are only 64 tRNA species,
then in a mixed population of tRNA's there would be a
total of 256 Ψ residues. No analytical procedure could have
detected the absence of two such residues. This is very
important to bear in mind as we discuss some of the other
modifications of tRNA in some other systems.

Regulation of Translation by tRNA Modification

The apparent function of one of the modifications of
tRNA was discovered independently by three different groups
of investigators. Most tRNA's are modified to various
extents on the base adjacent to the anticodon on the 3'OH
side. Gefter and Russell isolated an incompletely modified
tRNA^{Tyr} suppressor tRNA, synthesized after infection by
phage. This incompletely modified Su$^+_{III}$ tRNA^{Tyr} could be
charged with its cognate amino acid. However, it was
deficient in ribosomal binding reactions. The base adjacent
to the anticodon is an adenine which has three modifications:

149

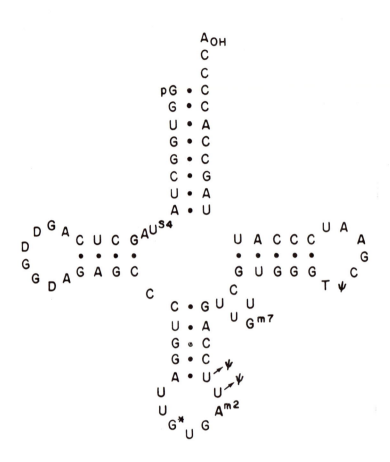

Fig. 1. *Schematic representation of the lack of modification by 2 Ψ in tRNA^His in a mutant of Salmonella.* For details see reference 9.

an N-6 isopentenyl group and a methylthio group in the three position. The degree of failure to attach to the ribosomes corresponds to the degree of lack of modification (10). Apparently the adenine must be totally modified for maximum efficiency. Hall *et al.* demonstrated essentially the same function for the modification of the base next to the anticodon (11). They prepared "isopentenyl deficient" tRNA by oxidation with permanganate. The unmodified product was ineffective in ribosomal attachment. Zachau and Thiebe have observed essentially the same phenomenon (12). One function, at least, of such modifications is now clear. Some factor for ribosomal binding must be anchored on that modified base.

Gefter exploited this observation for studying the *in vitro* synthesis of a specific protein by a partially modified tRNA. The clever strategy for this demonstration was as follows. The suppressor tRNA^{Tyr} was transcribed from phage DNA in a cell free system. This RNA is a suppressor of amber mutations in the gene coding for β-galactosidase. In an appropriate *in vitro* β-galactosidase synthesizing system the efficiency of the suppressor tRNA^{Tyr} could be enhanced fourfold by the addition of isopentenyl pyrophosphate which is a requisite for the post-transcriptional modification of the adenine adjacent to the anticodon (13).

It is difficult to visualize how the presence or absence of a non-reactive, hydrophobic group could effect or vitiate ribosomal attachment of a tRNA molecule which is hundreds of times larger than the modifying moiety. The difficulty of conceptualizing this stems from two sources. The original Watson-Crick hypothesis of interaction merely by base pairing of mRNA, tRNA and ribosomes still lingers in our minds. Slowly we identified numerous "factors" which we now recognize as requisite for initiation, ribosomal attachment and chain elongation. It is interesting that workers in this field are not bold enough to call these "factors" enzymes.

As I have pointed out elsewhere: "We are the slaves of classical organic chemistry, which concentrates on covalent linkages. We teach our students that enzymes make and break covalent bonds. Recognition of tRNA in some of its functions probably involves, of necessity, transient hydrophobic interactions, and for this reason progress in understanding mechanisms has been very slow. It is difficult to delineate "active sites" *etc.* in such weak inter-

actions" (14). Yet such a role for modification was predictable. "A second reason for methylation might be to contribute to the transfer function of tRNA, if the binding involves formation of hydrogen bonds then methylation could
affect the strength of these bonds" (1).

Wainwright *et al.* have demonstrated a regulatory function at the translational level for still another tRNA.
The biological system they exploited is the early chick
embryo which is incapable of synthesizing hemoglobin. If,
to an excised early embryonic disc, a population of transfer RNA's extracted from a later stage in the development
of the chick embryo is added, hemoglobin synthesis commences prematurely (15). Fractionation of the tRNA revealed
that the regulatory tRNA is a tRNA^{Ala}. It is highly probable that the tRNA^{Ala} which turns on hemoglobin synthesis
functions not in the synthesis of the hemoglobin itself
but rather in the synthesis of an enzyme involved in the
production of δ-amino levulinic acid, which is of course a
requisite for hemin synthesis. Whatever the mechanism, it
is obvious that this tRNA is translating prematurely a
pre-existing message. Shugart has reported still another
example of control by tRNA at translation. He isolated
from the apical part of the wheat leaf, which is essentially
senescent and does not grow, a population of tRNAs among
which a tRNA^{Phe} was found which has an incompletely modified
base next to the anticodon (16). Consequently, this tRNA
is defective in *in vitro* synthesis of poly U directed polyphenylalanine. Its deficiency in function is probably due
to improper binding to the ribosome as had been demonstrated
in other systems mentioned above.

tRNA Activity Unrelated to Protein Synthesis

Development of refined elution chromatographic systems
by the Oak Ridge group has had a burgeoning influence on
the study of variants of tRNA and their function. Thus,
Jacobson was enabled to study the population of tRNA's in a
vermilion mutant of Drosophila. An isoaccepting tRNA^{Tyr}
was observed in the tRNA population of this organism. In
a detailed study of this isoaccepting tRNA, Jacobson has
discovered a remarkable phenomenon. The isoaccepting
tRNA^{Tyr} has a function totally unrelated to protein synthesis.
It inhibits tryptophan pyrrolase, the first enzyme on the
pathway of pigment formation. Confirmatory evidence that
this function is totally unrelated to protein synthesis is

the activity of the tRNA whether it is charged or uncharged (17). This remarkable observation opens up a hitherto totally unexpected vista for tRNA functions, for it releases tRNA activity from the confines of the 64 anticodons. Indeed, it has been known for some time that in metazoa the number of tRNA species exceeds 64 by far. Often more than one isoaccepting tRNA responds to the same codon. The total number of isoaccepting tRNA's in any population is really unknown at the present time. We can predict that when more refined techniques are developed still larger numbers of isoaccepting tRNA's will be revealed. The variety of possible functions for such tRNA's must await research of the future.

Another function of a tRNA unrelated to mRNA-directed protein synthesis was discovered in Strominger's laboratory. In *Staphylococcus epidermis* there is a tRNA^{Gly} which, though is chargeable, can participate only in peptidoglycan synthesis (18).

Still another control function of tRNA unrelated to translation has been revealed, such as the inhibition of the first enzyme in the pathway of synthesis of the cognate amino acids. Thus, for example a tRNA^{Phe} inhibits the first enzyme on the aromatic pathway (19).

A 4S RNA has become implicated in the replication of RNA viruses via the reverse transcriptase (20,21). For example, Bishop in his studies of the mechanism of reverse transcription of the Rous sarcoma RNA, has purified the system sufficiently so that he can identify the necessary components. A chargeable but uncharged transfer RNA is an essential component of the system. It is apparently covalently bound to the emerging DNA through the 3' hydroxyl terminus of the transfer RNA. This transfer RNA is apparently a specific one, highly modified by methylation (22). This finding complements an earlier observation by Gantt who found that some tRNA methyltransferases are packaged in the Rous sarcoma virion (23). Also, Taylor, who has been studying the population of transfer RNA's themselves within the Rous sarcoma virion, observed a different population of transfer RNA's in a Rous sarcoma which is independent of a helper virus from the helper virus dependent Rous virion (24).

Hormonal Control of tRNA Structure

There are many lines of evidence indicating that

changes in the structure of tRNA's which result in novel
isoaccepting tRNA's can be the result *inter alia* of hormonal
activity. In our laboratory, we have demonstrated in several
systems that the tRNA methyltransferases are under hormonal
control. The most extensively studied are the tRNA methyltransferases in the normal uterus and in uteri of animals
which have undergone ovariectomy. In the uteri of ovariectomized animals the tRNA methyltransferase capacity falls
to one-half of that in the normal organ. This is not a
general reduction in the activity in all of the enzymes.
The patterns of diminution of activity of base specific
enzymes are individual (25). We have demonstrated similar
changes produced by hormonal activity in the metamorphosing
bull frog, *Rana catesbeiana*. Three days after the administration of thyroxine in physiological levels the transfer
RNA methylase capacity undergoes a profound diminution.
Two days later the enzyme activity returns to normal (26).

Changes in the transfer RNA methylating enzymes have
also been shown to be under hormonal control in mammary
tissue explants (27).

The administration of physiological doses of estradiol
to ovariectomized animals restores the transfer RNA methyltransferase activity to that in the normal uterus. There
are several lines of evidence demonstrating that the
structures themselves of transfer RNA are under hormonal
control. Thus for example, in the ovariectomized uterus a
novel isoaccepting tRNA^{Ser} appears (Fig. 2). Upon administration of physiological doses of estradiol this isoaccepting tRNA^{Ser} disappears from the population (Fig. 3) (25).
It should be emphasized that this is a reversible *qualitative*
effect of a hormone on a target organ.

*Modifications of tRNA Methylating Enzymes and of tRNA's
in Differentiating Systems*

Species specificity of tRNA structure prompted us to
suggest ten years ago that these modifications achieved
at great cost and energy must serve some species specific
function and we suggested that these should be studied in
systems with maximum expression of species individuality,
namely in differentiating systems. The first system we
studied was insects during metamorphosis. We observed
profound alterations in transfer RNA methylating capacity
during the eight day period in the pupae of *Tenebrio molitor*
prior to the emergence of the imago (28). Such studies have

154

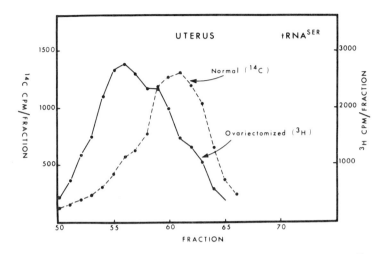

Fig. 2. *The appearance of a novel isoaccepting tRNA^{Ser} in the uterus of the ovariectomized sow.* For details see reference 25.

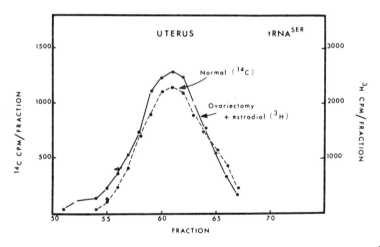

Fig. 3. *The disappearance of the novel isoaccepting tRNA^{Ser} from the uterus of the ovariectomized sow after administration of physiological doses of estradiol.* For details see reference 25.

been performed subsequently in a large variety of systems undergoing differentiation. These are listed in another review in this book (29). To our knowledge no exception has been found. In every differentiating tissue there are modifications in the transfer RNA methylating enzymes and invariably there is a concomitant change in the population of isoaccepting tRNA's. The most suggestive of these changes is one recently reported by Villee who finds that as early as in the two cell stage in the developing sea urchin embryo there is new synthesis of tRNA and this tRNA is newly methylated (30). We observed previously large changes in the tRNA methylating enzymes and in the methylated base pattern of tRNA's in later stages of the developing sea urchin embryo (31).

An intriguing modification of tRNA after its transcription has been discovered in reticulocytes by Farkas. Guanine is inserted into the primary sequence of nucleotides of a tRNA^{His}. The insertion is enzyme catalyzed and can be achieved *in vitro* (32). It will be interesting to determine the site of the insertion in the polynucleotide sequence.

tRNA and its Methylating Enzymes in Tumor Tissue

We were prompted to study the tRNA methyltransferases in tumor tissue by an observation by Magee and Farber. In the study of the carcinogenic activity of dimethylnitrosamine, Magee and Farber found that the carcinogen alkylates transfer RNA about ten times more than it alkylates DNA (33).

Examination of crude enzymes extracts from tumor tissue did indeed reveal hyperactivity of the tRNA methyltransferases in several tumors (34). These studies have been extended by many investigators and such hyperactivity has been observed in over 40 different tumors and cell lines transformed by oncogenic viruses. Tumors examined encompass the whole spectrum of etiology, various growth rates and transplanted as well as spontaneous tumors. They include the minimal deviation hepatomas with various growth rates and extents of de-differentiation (35).

Not only do the tRNA methyltransferases of tumor tissue differ quantitatively from those in normal tissue but it has been demonstrated recently by Dr. Sharma in our laboratory that they differ qualitatively as well (36).

After we observed that the tRNA methyltransferases are hyperactive in some tumors we hoped that any structural changes might be detected by the usual elution chromatographic

methods. We determined the elution profiles of every tRNA
species in the Novikoff hepatoma. We found three novel
tRNA's. These were that of tyrosine, histidine and aspara-
gine (37). Since then the populations of tRNA's have been
examined in a large number of tumors. Novel isoaccepting
tRNA's have been found in every tumor examined (35). Therefore, without exception there is a positive correlation between hyperactive transfer RNA methylases and the presence
of isoaccepting tRNA's in tumor tissue. Whether the hypermethylation is causal in the production of the isoaccepting
tRNA's is unknown. The isoaccepting tRNA's may have undergone different modification, or their primary sequence may
be different from those in the normal tissue counterpart.
Correlation between the methylation of tRNA's themselves
and the hyperactivity of the methylating enzymes themselves
in vitro is not established. There have been several reports in the literature demonstrating hypermethylation of
the tRNA's extracted from solid tumors (38). On the other
hand, there are reports that in transformed tissue cell
lines while the methylating capacity is high, no extensive
hypermethylation of the tRNA's themselves could be detected
(39). Minor component bases of tRNA's extracted from Morris
hepatomas have been recently analyzed in Randerath's laboratory and these authors report only slight changes in the
modification of the tRNA's from the tumor tissue (40). The
obvious shortcoming of all of these reported analyses is
that they are performed on the total population of tRNA's
extracted from mammalian tissue. Since as we stated earlier
many of the tRNA's in tumor cells are identical to those in
normal tissues and the number and quantity of atypical isoaccepting species are small, any changes in the isoaccepting
species in question would be masked during analysis by
the preponderance of the other, unchanged transfer RNA's.
We have pointed out at the beginning of this essay in
discussing the work of Bruce Ames that important, modulating transfer RNA's are often a small percentage of the
total population and therefore, changes among the isoaccepting species may not surface during analyses of the total
population of tRNAs.

The relatively small number of variant isoaccepting
species of tRNA's observed in tumor tissue is an enigma,
especially in view of the large excretion of tRNA components,
methylated purines, ψ, as well as degradation products of
erstwhile components of tRNA such as β aminoisobutyric acid

derived from thymine (41), in the urine of human patients with cancer and in the urine of tumor bearing animals. As has been suggested recently by Sheid, hypermethylated tRNA's may become functionally inactive and therefore, they are eliminated rapidly (42). This would explain the origin of the large excretion of tRNA components and the absence of highly methylated tRNA's from some tumors and transformed cell lines. (However, were this the case the novel iso-accepting tRNA's found in tumor tissues would be randomly distributed among the whole population of tRNA's and the contrary is the experimental finding: the isoaccepting tRNA's isolated from a given tumor are always the same species.) It is certain that these paradoxes will be re-solved with more refined analyses of specific tRNA's and also with the emergence of heretofore unknown functions of some of the modified tRNA's.

Presented by Ernest Borek

References

1. Borek, E. The methylation of transfer RNA: mechanism and function. Cold Spring Harbor Symp. 28: 139 (1963).
2. Fleissner, E. Personal Communication. (1962).
3. Srinivasan, P.R. and E. Borek. The species variation of RNA methylase. Proc. Nat. Acad. Sci. 49: 529 (1963).
4. Von Ehrenstein, G. and F. Lipmann. Experiments on hemoglobin biosynthesis. Proc. Nat. Acad. Sci. USA 47: 941 (1961).
5. Hunter, A.R. and R.J. Jackson. Miscoding by *E. Coli* tRNA's for methionine, cysteine and valine in the synthesis of rabbit globin. Europ. J. Biochem. 15: 381 (1970).
6. Mandel, L.R. and E. Borek. The source of methyl group for the thymine of RNA. Biochem. Biophys. Res. Commun. 6: 138 (1961).
7. Borek, E., A. Ryan and J. Rockenbach. Nucleic acid metabolism in relation to the lysogenic phenomenon. J. Bacteriol. 69: 460 (1955).
8. Ames, B.N. and P.E. Hartman. The histidine operon. Cold Spring Harbor Symp. 28: 349 (1963).

9. Singer, C.E., G.E., R. Cortese and B.N. Ames. Mutant tRNA^{His} ineffective in repression and lacking 2 pseudouridine modifications. Nature New Biol. 238: 72 (1972).

10. Gefter, M.L. and R.L. Russell. Role of modifications in transfer RNA: A modified base affecting ribosomal binding. J. Mol. Biol. 39: 145 (1969).

11. Fittler, E. and R.H. Hall. Selective modification of yeast seryl tRNA and its effect on the acceptance and binding functions. Biochem. Biophys. Res. Commun. 25: 441 (1966).

12. Thiebe, R. and H.G. Zachau. A specific modification next to the anticodon of phenylalanine transfer ribonucleic acid. Europ. J. Biochem. 5: 546 (1968).

13. Zubay, G., L. Cheong and M. Gefter. The DNA-directed cell-free synthesis of a biologically active transfer RNA: Su$^+$ III tyrosyl tRNA. Proc. Nat. Acad. Sci. USA 69: 2195 (1971).

14. Borek, E. Recognition sites in tRNA. J. Cell. Physiol. 74: 161 (1969).

15. Wainwright, S.D., L.K. Wainwright and H.M. Tsay. Regulation of hemoglobin synthesis in the blood islands of chick blastodiscs: tentative identification of the stimulatory transfer RNA as a minor alanine specific species. Canad. J. Biochem. 50: 1158 (1972).

16. Shugart, L. A possible age related modification of phenylalanine transfer RNA from wheat tissue. Expt. Geront. 7: 251 (1972).

17. Jacobson, K.B. Role of isoacceptor transfer RNA as an enzyme inhibitor: Effect on tryptophan pyrrolase on *Drosophila*. Nature 231: 17 (1971).

18. Stewart, T.S., R.J. Roberts and J.L. Strominger. Novel species of tRNA. Nature 230: 36 (1971).

19. Duda, E., M. Staub, P. Venetianer and G. Denes. Interaction between tRNA^{Phe} and the allosteric first enzyme of the aromatic amino acid biosynthetic pathway. Biochem. Biophys. Res. Commun. 32: b92 (1968).

20. Manly, K.F., D.F. Smoler, E. Bromfield and D. Baltimore. sRNA requirement for reverse transcriptase. J. Virol. 7: 106 (1971).

21. Rosenthal, L.J. and P.C. Zamecnick. Minor base composition of "70S-associated" 4s RNA from avian myeloblastosis virus. Proc. Nat. Acad. Sci. USA 70: 865 (1973).

22. Faras, A.J., M.M. Best, J.M. Taylor, W.E. Levinson, H.M. Goodman and J.M. Bishop. DNA polymerase of Rous

sarcoma virus: identification of RNA primer molecule required for initiation of DNA synthesis. J. Virol. (in press).

23. Gantt, R., K. Stromberg and F. Montes de Oca. Specific RNA methylase associated with avian myeloblastosis virus. Nature 234: 35 (1971).

24. Wang, S., R.M. Kothari, M. Taylor and P. Hung. Transfer RNA activities of Rous sarcoma and Rous associated viruses. Nature New Biol. 242: 133 (1973).

25. Sharma, O.K. and E. Borek. Hormonal effect on transfer ribonucleic acid methylases and on serine transfer ribonucleic acid. Biochem. 9: 2507 (1970).

26. Pillinger, D.J., W.K. Paik and E. Borek. The tRNA methylases during thyroxine-induced differentiation in bull frog tadpoles. J. Endocrinol. 49: 547 (1971).

27. Turkington, R.W. and M. Riddle. Transfer RNA methylating enzymes in mammary carcinoma cells. Cancer Res. 30: 650 (1970).

28. Baliga, B.S., P.R. Srinivasan and E. Borek. Changes in the tRNA methylating enzymes during insect metamorphosis. Nature 208: 555 (1965).

29. Kerr, S.J. Control of tRNA methyltransferase activity by competing enzyme systems. Chapter 5, this conference.

30. O'Melia, F. and C.A. Villee. *De novo* synthesis of transfer RNA and 5S RNA in cleaving sea urchin embryos. Nature 239: 51 (1972).

31. Sharma, O.K., L. Loeb and E. Borek. Transfer RNA methylases during sea urchin embryogenesis. Biochim. Biophys. Acta 240: 558 (1971).

32. Hankins, W.D. and W.R. Farkas. Guanylation of transfer RNA by rabbit reticulocytes. Biochim. Biophys. Acta 213: 77 (1970).

33. Magee, P.N. and E. Farber. Toxic liver injury and carcinogenesis methylation of rat liver nucleic acids by dimethylnitrosamine *in vivo*. Biochem. J. 83: 114 (1962).

34. Tsutsui, E., P.R. Srinivasan and E. Borek. tRNA methylases in tumors of animal and human origin. Proc. Nat. Acad. Sci. USA 56: 1003 (1966).

35. Borek, E. Introduction. Cancer Research 31: 596 (1971).

36. Sharma, O.K. Differences in the transfer RNA methyltransferases from normal rat liver and Novikoff hepatoma. Biochim. Biophys. Acta 299: 415 (1973).

37. Baliga, B.D., E. Borek, I.B. Weinstein and P.R. Srinivasan. Differences in the transfer RNAs of normal liver and Novikoff hepatoma. Proc. Nat. Acad. Sci. USA 62: 899 (1969).

38. Borek, E. and S.J. Kerr. Atypical transfer RNA's and their origin in neoplastic cells. Advances in Cancer Res. 15: 163 (1972).

39. Klagsbrun, M. The contrast between the methylation of transfer ribonucleic acid *in vivo* and *in vitro* by normal and SV40 transformed 3T3 cells. J. Biol. Chem. 247: 7443 (1972).

40. Randerath, E., L.S.Y. Chia, J.B. Williams, H.P. Morris and K. Randerath. Comparative studies on liver and hepatoma tRNA. Federation Proc. Abs. 32: 653 (1973).

41. Nielsen, H.R., E. Borek, K. Sjølin and K. Nyholm. Dual origin of β-aminoisobutyric acid, a thymine catabolite. Acta Path. Microbiol. Scand. Section A 80: 687 (1972).

42. Sheid, B. Personal Communication.

THE USE OF REGULATORY "MUTANTS" IN THE ANALYSIS OF
CELL-HORMONE INTERACTION

Gordon M. Tomkins

Introduction

Vertebrate hormones regulate physiological processes
in fully differentiated cells and control numerous aspects
of development. In relatively recent years, the broad
outlines of the molecular bases of the action of a number
of hormones have become clear although, of course, a great
deal remains to be discovered about specific details.
However, many unresolved questions concerning hormone
action extend well beyond the confines of this subject and
into important unknown areas of general biology. This
state of affairs derives from the fact that the two major
cellular sites of hormone action appear to be the cell
membrane and the chromosomes. Since both of these complex
structures are relatively poorly understood, it seems probable that studies of hormone action will contribute much
to the understanding of membrane and chromosome structure.
Conversely, a more detailed knowledge of these entities is
required for a deeper understanding of the hormones themselves.
     In the present discussion I shall present some of our
recent studies illustrating the use of quasi-genetic techniques to explore these aspects of cell-hormone interaction. Most of the work in our laboratory has been con-
cerned with the mechanism of glucocorticoid induction of
tyrosine aminotransferase in cultured rat hepatoma cells
(1). From this work, and a multitude of studies in different laboratories, it appears as though this process can
serve as a model for the molecular action of all the steroid hormones. In brief, biologically active corticoids
penetrate the membranes of target cells and form non-co-
valent associations with high-affinity specific receptor
protein molecules primarily located in the cytoplasm. The

receptors are probably allosteric proteins (2) and interaction between hormone and receptor either induces or
stabilizes structural changes in the latter, permitting
the receptor-steroid complex to localize in the nucleus
(3), associating with a large number of specific high affinity DNA-containing acceptor sites (4). This interaction brings about an accumulation of messenger RNA molecules coding for specific proteins, the synthesis of which
alters the cell phenotype in response to the hormonal
stimulation.

This sequence of events has been delineated largely
by biochemical studies carried out either in intact cells
or in cell extracts. To verify the pathway as well as to
get more detailed insight into the interactions between
the receptor-steroid complexes and nuclear acceptor sites,
it seemed desirable to use biological as well as biochemical approaches. For this reason, we have been studying a
number of cell lines derived from mouse immunocytes. The
growth of these cells is inhibited by the glucocorticoids
and treatment with these hormones ultimately causes cell
death (5,6). It seems likely that this phenomenon is
related to the immunosuppressive action of the steroids
and forms the basis for the therapeutic use of these hormones in leukemia. Although circumstantial evidence suggests that the glucocorticoids induce macromolecules
which somehow cause cell death (7) the precise mechanism
of killing is not known. Nevertheless, it is possible to
take advantage of steroid-induced cell killing in order to
obtain steroid-insensitive cell lines.

Materials and Methods

All the techniques used in these studies have been
described in recent publications from our laboratory and
are referred to in the appropriate sections of the text.

Results and Discussion

Figure 1 (8) illustrates that physiological concentrations of the synthetic glucocorticoid, dexamethasone, kills
"wild type" cultured Balb/c mouse lymphoma cells of the
S49 line. In this experiment, cell death was measured by
the loss of the ability of treated cells to form colonies

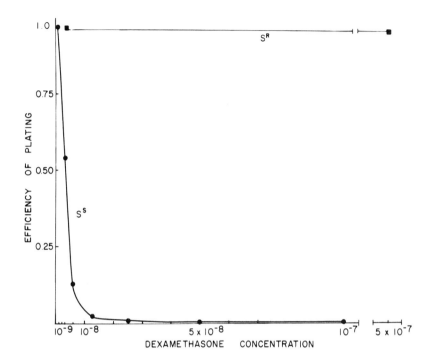

Fig. 1. *Growth response of steroid-sensitive and resistant clones to dexamethason.* Appropriate dilutions of sensitive (●) and resistant (■) clones were plated in the presence of the indicated concentrations of dexamethasone. The number of clones per plate was counted at the end of ten days. The efficiency of plating shown is the average of five identical plates, (from (8)).

165

in soft agar overlying a feeder layer of mouse embryo fibroblasts. Whereas the vast majority of treated cells cannot form colonies, an occasional steroid-resistant clone is seen. Figure 1 also shows the effect of increasing steroid concentrations on the colony-forming ability of such steroid-resistant colonies. Clearly cells derived from these clones are extremely resistant to the killing actions of dexamethasone. Further experiments have shown that steroid resistance is maintained even when resistant cells are grown for prolonged periods in the absence of dexamethasone.

Luria-Delbruck fluctuation tests indicate that the emergence of the presence of the selective agent at a rate of approximately 3×10^{-6} per cell per generation (9). These properties are consistent either with a mutation or a spontaneous heritable variation. To attempt to differentiate between these possibilities, we have examined the effects of different mutagenic agents on the frequency of steroid-resistant variants. Three treatments were used: X-ray, 9-aminoacridine and nitrosoguanadine. Each of them significantly increased the frequency of steroid resistance, suggesting that the transition from sensitivity to resistance might be mutational in origin. Needless to say this conclusion cannot be formly drawn in the absence of a demonstrated amino acid substitution in a particular protein. However, a mutational basis for the emergence of steroid-resistance seems a very likely possibility.

Since glucocorticoid killing is probably attributable to the induction of "lethal macromolecules" it seems likely that the initial steps in cell-hormone interaction in lymphoma cells should be the same as the steps outlined for the induction of tyrosine aminotransferase synthesis in cultured hepatoma cells. If this is true, then the steroid-resistant lymphoma cells could be defective in any of the early steps in hormone action. For example, certain cells should be defective in steroid receptor activity. We call this predicted phenotype, "R^-". Certain colonies might retain normal steroid-binding activity (R^+) but be unable to transfer the receptor-steroid complex to the nucleus. We disignate this predicted class of variants "N^-". Finally, cells might become resistant for any of a variety of reasons which render the reactions subsequent to the nuclear binding step inactivate. We call this phenotype "deathless" and designate it as "D^-".

In order to classify a given steroid-resistant variant according to the steps in hormone action, a crude cell fractionation method was devised in which total hormone uptake is measured first. This is followed by cell rupture by freezing and thawing, and then separation of the crude nuclear fraction from the soluble fraction by differential centrifugation.

Using this technique (9), 66 independently isolated steroid-resistant clones were analyzed. Of them, about 80% were unable to concentrate the radioactive dexamethasone suggesting they were defective in the initial steroid receptor interaction, $i.e.$, they were R⁻. This impression was confirmed by preparing cell-free extracts of such cells and measuring the ability of particle-free supernatants to form receptor-steroid complexes. An experiment of this type is illustrated in Figure 2 (8). It can be seen that the wild-type cells contain receptor molecules which associate with high affinity with the added dexamethasone whereas resistant cells classified at R⁻ on the basis of the whole cell experiments described above do not contain such receptor activity. About 2/3 of the remaining 20% of the receptor-containing (R⁺) resistant clones, contained receptor steroid complexes which migrated to the nucleus. These clones were therefore D⁻. A third class of variants which formed receptor-steroid complexes, but in which these complexes failed to associate with the nucleus (N⁻) was also found.

These data conform closely to the predications of the model for the early steps in cell-steroid interaction presented above. They are consistent with the idea that receptor molecules are required for the glucocorticoid effects and that the receptor-steroid complex must associate with nuclear sites. The presence of D⁻ cells also illustrates that this interaction although necessary is not sufficient to produce the killing effect implying that subsequent events presumably involving the induction of macromolecular synthesis must ensue before cell death takes place. The existence of these various classes of steroid-resistant variants holds out the hope that more detailed chemical analyses of the molecular basis of the resistance could lead to a fuller understanding of cell-steroid interactions.

It should also be possible to use somatic cell hybridization procedures to determine the number of complementa-

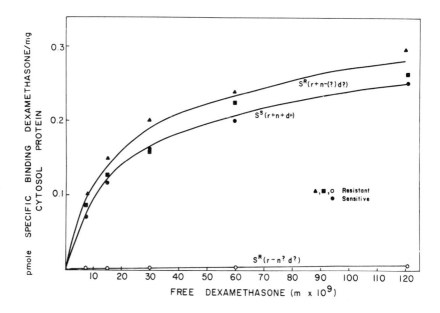

Fig. 2. *Specific steroid binding by extracts of steroid-sensitive and representative resistant lymphoma clones.* Fresh cell pellets were homogenized at $2°C$ in hypotonic buffer (20 mM Ticine, 2 mM $CaCl_2$, 1 mM $MgCl_2$ pH 7.8) and spun at 100,000 x g for one hour. These particle-free supernatants were incubated at $2°C$ for 90 min with the indicated concentration of (^3H) dexamethasone (35 Ci/mole) with and without 5 x 10^{-5} M unlabeled dexamethasone as competitor. The differnce between these is plotted as specific binding. Values are the average of 3 to 4 determinations. Protein concentrations were determined by the method of Lowrey, et al. (1951). The resistant clones were either r^- (0) or r^+. One of the latter (▲) was shown to be r^+n^- by the technique described in the legend to Fig. 2, (from ref. 8).

tion groups, and therefore the number of functional elements, involved in the overall interation of hormones with their specific target cells. Some experiments of this type have already been carried out (7) and the results indicate that the D^+ phenotype is dominant to deathlessness, suggesting that glucocorticoids do induce macromolecules leading to cell killing.

In addition to the hormones whose actions are mediated by cytoplasmic receptors, there are biological effectors which function by associating with specific membrane receptors. These substances include a large number of hormones as well as many drugs. Genetic studies with the S49 lymphoma line can also be used to study these interactions because dibutyryl cyclic AMP, like the steroid hormones, leads to cell killing when added to the culture medium. By growing populations of S49 cells in increasing concentrations of the cyclic nucleotide, we have derived populations resistant to millimolar concentrations of dibutyryl cyclic AMP (10). As might be expected, "wildtype" S49 cells are also growth-inhibited by agents which evoke the production of cyclic AMP (cholera toxin, epinephrine, prostagladin E_1) or which inhibit its destruction (theophylline). Cells selected for resistance to dibutyryl cyclic AMP-insensitive cells contain much lower quantities of cyclic AMP-sensitive protein kinase and its associated regulatory subunit, than wild type cells. We have begun to use these cells to analyze the biochemical basis of norepinephrine-induced enzyme synthesis (11). This sympathomimetic amine induces the synthesis of cyclic AMP phosphodiesterase in S49 cells (12); however, only in wildtype cyclic AMP-sensitive cells, and not in the kinase-deficient resistant cells. Although indirect, these studies indicate that the cAMP-activated kinase is involved in cyclic AMP-mediated enzyme induction, as well as in the other aspects of cyclic nucleotide action.

Summary

1. S49 mouse lymphoma cells are killed by glucocorticoids such as dexamethasone.
2. Stably resistant variants can be isolated.
3. Resistance arises at random with a rate of about 3×10^{-6} per cell per generation but this rate can be

augmented by a variety of mutagens.
4. Three phenotypes of steroid resistance have been detected, corresponding to the early steps in steroid hormone action detected by biochemical means.
5. Cyclic AMP and hormones which stimulate its production also kill S49 cells.
6. Cells resistant to these agents may also be isolated and used to study hormone and drug action.
7. Genetic studies of this type should help biochemical investigations into the mechanisms of hormone action.

Presented by Gordon M. Tomkins, Department of Biochemistry and Biophysics, University of California, San Francisco, San Francisco, California 94143.

References

1. Baxter, J.D., G.G. Rousseau, S.J. Higgins and G.M. Tomkins. Mechanism of glucocorticoid hormone action and of regulation of gene expression in cultured mammalian cells. In: The Biochemistry of Gene Expression in Higher Organisms, J.K. Pollak and J.W. Lee, (Editors). Australia and New Zealand Book Company, Sydney, pp. 206-224.
2. Samuels, H.H. and G.M. Tomkins. The relation of steroid structure to enzyme induction in hepatoma tissue culture cells. J. Mol. Biol. 52: 57 (1970).
3. Baxter, J.D. and G.M. Tomkins. The relationship between glucocorticoid binding and tyrosine aminotransferase induction in hepatoma tissue culture cells. Proc. Nat. Acad. Sci. USA 65: 709-715 (1970).
4. Baxter, J.D., G.G. Rousseau, M.C. Benson, R.L. Garcea, J. Ito and G.M. Tomkins. Role of DNA and specific cytoplasmic receptors in glucocorticoid action. Proc. Nat. Acad. Sci. USA 69: 1892 (1972).
5. Gehring, U., B. Mohit and G.M. Tomkins. Interaction of glucocorticoids with cultured lymphoid cells. Proceedings of the Fourth International Congress of Endocrinology. Excerpta Medica. In press.
6. Rosenau, W., J.D. Baxter, G.G. Rousseau and G.M. Tomkins. Mechanism of resistance to steroids: glucocorticoid receptor defect in lymphoma cells. Nature

New Biol. 237: 20 (1972).

7. Gehring, U., B. Mohit and G.M. Tomkins. Gluco-corticoid action on hybrid clones derived from cultured myeloma and lymphoma cell lines. Proc. Nat Acad. Sci. USA 69: 3124 (1972).

8. Sibley, C.H., U. Gehring, H. Bourne and G.M. Tomkins. Hormonal control of cellular growth. In: Control of Proliferation in Animal Cells, B. Clarkson and R. Baserga, (Editors). Cold Spring Harbor Laboratory.

9. Sibley, C.H. and G.M. Tomkins. Frequency of resistant variants in a glucocorticoid-sensitive population of cultured mouse lymphoma cells. Abstract. Genetics 74: s253 (1973).

10. Daniel, V., G. Litwack and G.M. Tomkins. Induction of cytolysis of cultured lymphoma cells by adenosine 3': 5'-cyclic monophosphate and the isolation of resistant variants. Proc. Nat. Acad. Sci. USA 70: 76 (1973).

11. Daniel, V., H.R. Bourne and G.M. Tomkins. Altered metabolism and endogenous cyclic AMP in cultured cells deficient in cyclic-AMP binding proteins. Nature New Biol. 244: 167 (1973).

12. Bourne, H.R., G.M. Tomkins and S. Dion. Regulation of phosphodiesterase synthesis: requirement for cyclic AMP-dependent protein kinase. Science. In press.

DNA DAMAGE AND REPAIR DURING CARCINOGENESIS

Emmanuel Farber and D.S.R. Sarma

It is evident that the planet earth is basically a
hostile environment for all living organisms, including man.
Among the long list of hazards, from the point of view of
cancer, are not only various forms of radiation but also an
increasing number of viruses and a growing list of chemicals.
Of the latter, although by far the greater number are associated with some activites of man, be it some cultural
pattern or some modern day industrial operation, there is
also a significant number of naturally-occurring chemicals.
We are now becoming more aware of the latter, especially as
they may relate to some special geographic incidence of one
or another form of cancer. In addition, we must not over-
look hazardous chemicals generated in the body from normal
small precursor molecules. Outstanding among the latter
are the nitrosamines and nitrosamides, so relatively easily
formed in the gastrointestinal tract from nitrites and
secondary amines (1).

The varied chemical nature of the many carcinogens
presented for years a baffling barrier to any reasonable
hypothesis of their mode of action. In an early attempt to
present a working hypothesis, Haddow suggested many years
ago that carcinogens may be alkylating agents or converted
to such active molecules by the body. Work during the
past 15 years in a few laboratories, spearheaded by the
outstanding work of the Millers (2), is providing increas-
ingly solid evidence in favor of this thesis. The majority
of the chemicals so far studied are either electrophilic
reactants *per se* or are converted to such active derivatives
called ultimate carcinogens, by enzymes, usually microsomal
in distribution, in the appropriate target tissues. In at
least some instances (*i.e.*, some nitrosamides), their re-
activity is enhanced by cysteine, glutathione or possibly
some other SH compounds (3).

The two major conceptual advances in chemical carcinogenesis made during the past few years have been (a) the
discovery of enzyme activation of most procarcinogens to
the reactive ultimate carcinogens (2) and (b) the chemical
interaction of the activated molecule with a variety of
tissue nucleophiles including DNA, RNA and protein (2,4,5).

(a) The enzymatic activation of procarcinogens is well
established and needs only a passing reference. It must be
emphasized that enzyme induction by drugs was discovered by
the Millers and Conney in their studies of the effects of
3-methylcholanthrene on azo dye metabolism. In addition,
the occurrence of biological N-hydroxylation of aromatic
amines was also discovered in the same laboratory. The
study of nitrosamines in Magee's laboratory (6) and studies
with ethionine by Stekol (7) and ourselves (8) offer
further examples of enzyme activation to electrophiles by
target tissues.

(b) Early in the post war period, Miller and Miller
discovered that carcinogens bind to tissue proteins. Subsequently, this binding property was extended to RNA and
DNA. Today it is evident that virtually all chemical carcinogens, when activated, interact with all the major tissue macromolecules. In proteins, several amino acids,
including histidine, methionine, cysteine, tryptophane and
tyrosine, react with different carcinogens. In DNA and RNA,
the major known sites are N-7 and C-8 of guanine. However,
many other reactive sites have been described, such as N-3
and 0-6 of guanine, N-1, N-3 and N-7 of adenine and N-1 of
cytosine (9).

The patterns of reaction with different RNA's vary
with the carcinogen. Some, *i.e.*, ethionine and to a lesser
degree 2-acetylaminofluorene (AAF) react most avidly with
tRNA. Others, such as nitrosamines, seem to be less selective.

Thus, not unexpectedly, the production of highly reactive derivatives of carcinogens leads to chemical interaction with a whole spectrum of target sites in all major
cell constituents. How can one intelligently select those
reactions that are most relevant to carcinogenesis and in
what manner are they relevant?

Before any rational attempt can be made at such a
judgement, we must look briefly at some of the biological
characteristics of carcinogenesis (10): (a) It is now
widely accepted that the carcinogenic process in most tis-

sues is a multistep process. This has been appreciated for many years both from human and experimental studies. A major advance occurred in 1940 with the separation of the carcinogenic process in the skin into an initial rapid irreversible step, called initiation and a complex subsequent process called promotion. The latter is much more aptly called neoplastic development or evolution. The most important discovery was the finding that initiation was a property of carcinogens while the subsequent development or evolution could be accelerated by non-carcinogenic promoting agents or co-carcinogens as well as by carcinogens. Subsequently, an increasing body of evidence with many different carcinogens in many different systems indicates the wide applicability of this principle, although no model developed yet is as elegant as is the skin model.

(b) With models in which carcinogenesis is initiated by a brief exposure to the carcinogen, there is often an apparent eclipse period of weeks before any obvious cellular changes can be detected. Thus, whatever the essential nature of initiation, it must have the property of a relatively long memory component. DNA is most easily handled conceptually in this context.

These considerations, together with the following two, favor the suggestion that DNA may be a major probable target in carcinogenesis: (c) carcinogens, if properly activated, are mutagenic in bacteriophage, bacteria or even in some eukaryotes; and (d) patients with a rare disease, xeroderma pigmentosum, associated with a very high incidence of skin cancer, often show defects in repair of ultra-violet light induced or of some carcinogen induced DNA damage.

What is the nature of the damage to DNA induced by carcinogens and what are the patterns of repair?

Four basic approaches are now available to monitor damage and repair of DNA in eukaryotic cells:

(a) the production or removal of the chemical alterations in DNA, be they pyrimidine dimer, bound forms of a chemical or some chemical consequences of the latter;

(b) the availability of new groups, such as phosphate groups, to enzymatic attack upon rupture of a DNA strand;

(c) the incorporation of deoxynucleotide precursors or analogues, such as bromodeoxyuridine, into DNA not actively engaged in its own replication ("unscheduled DNA synthesis");

(d) measurement of the average size of the DNA, either

175

as a single-stranded (alkaline sucrose gradient) or double-stranded (neutral sucrose gradient) molecule.

Most of the initial work on the study of DNA damage by carcinogens has involved unscheduled DNA synthesis, either in human lymphocytes (11) or in other cells *in vitro*, both normal and disease (12). These studies have clearly shown that most active forms of carcinogens can induce DNA repair, presumably as a consequence of damage. With these various cell systems, which by and large don't show metabolic activation of many procarcinogens to the active moieties (except for some polycyclic aromatic hydrocarbons), only ultimate carcinogens or carcinogens not requiring conversion to an active form damage DNA. This retricts the use very seriously. This defect can be circumvented in some instances by adding to the medium a preparation of liver microsomes plus suitable coenzymes (NADP) *etc.*, to carry out the activation. The active moieties can then penetrate the intact cells and interact with the DNA, *etc.*

Although this approach is interesting and useful, it is not directly applicable as yet to the study of carcinogenesis, since the systems used are not appropriate for the induction of neoplastic transformation by most chemicals.

It is mainly for this reason that we began to explore other systems which would have a greater obvious relevance to carcinogenesis. The liver proved to be amenable to such studies. A method was developed in our laboratory to monitor relative size of DNA using sedimentation velocity in sucrose gradients. This is basically a method first described for *E. coli* DNA that was subsequently used for cells in tissue culture (13,14). After appropriate modifications and changes, it has become extremely useful in giving us a new prespective on DNA damage and repair and its possible importance in liver carcinogenesis.

During the initial survey of many hepatotoxic agents including carcinogens and non-carcinogens, certain patterns of damage and especially repair have begun to become evident. All the various compounds tested fall into one of four categories: (a) compounds inducing single strand damage in liver DNA that is relatively rapidly repaired (4 to 72 hours) (Table I). These agents are either carcinogens for organs other than the liver, (except under special circumstances), or are not known to be carcinogens for want of testing. One example of a special circumstance

TABLE I

Compounds Inducing Liver DNA Damage (Single Strand)
With Repair Within 4 to 72 Hours

N-methyl-N-nitrosourea	Ethylmethanesulfonate
N-methyl-N-nitroso-N'- nitroguanidine	4-nitroquinoline-N-oxide
Methylnitrosourethane	4-hydroxyaminoquinoline-N-oxide
Methylmethanesulfonate	Camptothecin
N-ethyl-N-nitrosourea	Bleomycin*

*Results of R. Cox (personal communication)

177

applies to hycanthone and is particularly interesting. This compound intercalates into DNA and is not carcinogenic for mouse liver following a single administration. However, when used in mice with schistosomiasis, an important disease in which it is used in its treatment, it has been found to induce liver neoplasms (15). Thus, there is a strong possibility that at least some of the compounds in group (a) may prove to be carcinogenic for liver when tested under some special circumstances.

(b) Compounds inducing single-strand damage in liver DNA that is only slowly repaired (a few days to weeks) (Table II). These compounds are almost all liver carcinogens.

(c) Compounds inducing double-strand as well as single strand damage to liver DNA (Table III). These compounds may show slow or rapid repair of both types of damage, although so far the double-strand damage seems to be more rapidly repaired than is the single-strand.

(d) Hepatotoxic compounds that induce liver damage but do not seem to cause *primary* damage to DNA (Table IV). Some damage to DNA may appear with these agents but this is late and a probable consequence of cell death with degradation and removal of the dead liver cells. Since DNA is degraded as part of the tissue and cellular repair processes, it is important to stress that the study of DNA damage and repair must be done under conditions in which there is no development of irreversible loss of cell integrity.

The above findings have suggested a new hypothesis of the initiation event(s) in cancer induction - the induction of double-strand damage to DNA with its attendant high probability of errors in the subsequent repair process. According to current views of DNA damage and repair (16,17), mechanisms are available for the faithful reconstruction of the damaged single-strand so long as the complementary strand remains intact. Thus, induction of single-strand damage is probably followed in most instances by extensive or complete repair. Since so much of the DNA in the eukaryote is non-functional at any physiologic state in an adult organ, one would imagine that this type of damage would have only few if any functional consequences under most circumstances. This is valid in a population of cells that are quiescent and not undergoing continuous proliferation, such as the liver. However, if DNA replication is induced before repair of the single-strand damage is com-

TABLE II

Compounds Inducing Liver DNA Damage (Single Strand)
With Slow Repair

Dimethylnitrosamine	2-acetylaminofluorene
Methylazoxymethanol acetate	N-nitrosopiperidine
Diethylnitrosamine	N-N-dinitrosopiperazine

TABLE III

Compounds Inducing Double Strand Damage
to Liver DNA

N-hydroxy-2-acetylamino- fluorene	Nitrosodihydrouracil
N-acetoxy-2-acetylamino- fluorene	3-hydroxyxanthine
N-nitrosomorpholine	Hycanthone methanesulfonate

TABLE IV

Heptotoxic Compounds Inducing No Obvious
Primary Damage to Liver DNA

Cycloheximide	Galactosamine
Morpholine	α-amanitine
Piperidine	Isopentenyladenosine
Piperazine	Nitrosocitrulline
Cyclophosphamide	

plete, then a new aspect of the process appears - how does the cell replicate its DNA when one or more parts are defective? One way is to use the newly replicated complementary copy of the other strand by a process called recombination repair (postreplication repair). This has been worked out to some degree in bacteria but not well in eukaryotes.

Double-strand breaks pose even greater problems if these are truly occurring at the same relative position in each of the two strands of the DNA and one or more bases are removed in each strand. How such a lesion is repaired is not known. However, some "sealing" of the break unquestionably occurs. We feel that the repair of such lesions by whatever mechanism might very well lead to some loss of historical continuity in the base sequence of that part of the DNA and therefore to some error-prone repair.

According to our current views, the repair of at least some of the double-strand breaks or the occurrence of an episode of DNA replication before a single-strand break is repaired could well induce permanent biochemical lesions in the DNA of susceptible cells. This is a "simple" hypothesis for *initiation* that is attractive (18). This could account for the patterns observed so far and for the observations that partial hepatectomy may enable a single exposure to a carcinogen to induce liver cancer with agents that normally require longer exposure to the same agent for neoplastic development (*see*, 19).

It should be emphasized that such lesions of DNA are probably not sufficient to induce cancer. They merely are enabling phenomena, essential but not sufficient for carcinogenesis. The many events occurring during "promotion" including selective cell proliferation must occur subsequent to the initiation event(s). A knowledge of these events is essential if we are to truly understand how lesions of DNA fit into the carcinogenic process, assuming that they play some role at all.

One aspect of DNA damage and repair that has not been mentioned yet but one that could play an important role in the neoplastic process is the interaction of the carcinogen with selective aspects of DNA. Do carcinogens react randomly or is there a reproducible and directed pattern? Recent work in our laboratory indicates that one carcinogen, dimethylnitrosamine, might interact with some portions of the DNA much more avidly than with other portions. The im-

portant questions now become: if confirmed, does this sel-
ectivity apply only to the primary damage or is there also
selective rates of repair for the same type of chemical damage for different segments of the DNA? There are no
straightforward ways to explore these problems today. However, there are approaches that are being explored.

Before concluding, it is important to touch on one
further aspect of repair - *in vivo* versus *in vitro* and
"resting" versus proliferating cells. Most of the work *in
vitro* is with cells in culture. Here, by and large, most
damaging agents, whether carcinogenic or not, do pretty
much the same degree of damage and repair in about the same
time period - 12 to 24 hours. It is already evident that
this is far from the case *in vivo* in a resting organ such
as liver (14). Obviously, since neoplasia occurs in the
latter with chemicals, it is especially important to study
this if one hopes to relate molecular events to biology as
they concern cancer.

Problems such as the exact chemical nature of the damage with different carcinogens, the enzymes involved in
various types of repair, the rate limiting steps in each
type of repair and the alteration of the rate of limiting
step by inducing agents, are but a few of the key questions
that must be answered if we are to have any understanding
of how DNA is damaged and repaired. Since so many environmental agents and influences, including carcinogens, interact with DNA, this has potential importance not only for
cancer but for our understanding of other fundamental processes in biology including evolution.

In conclusion, we are optimistic that the newer approaches now being developed for the study of DNA damage and
repair in the tissues of an intact animal under the influence of carcinogens may offer new insights into phases of
cancer and carcinogenesis that have hitherto been unexplor-
ed. Hopefully, new ideas concerning the molecular mechanisms of carcinogenesis may develop.

---

*Presented by Emmanuel Farber, American Cancer Society Re-
search Professor. The authors' research was supported in
part by research grants from the National Institutes of
Health (CA-10439, CA-12218 and AM-14882), American Cancer
Society (BC-7N) and an institutional grant to Temple University from the American Cancer Society.*

References

1. Lijinsky, W. and S.S. Epstein. Nitrosamines as environmental carcinogens. Nature 225: 21 (1970).
2. Miller, J.A. Carcinogenesis by chemicals: an overview-G.H.A. Clowes Memorial Lecture. Cancer Res. 30: 559 (1970).
3. Lawley, P.D. and C.J. Thatcher. Methylation of deoxyribonucleic acid in cultured mamalian cells by N-methyl-N'-nitro-N-nitrosoguanidine. Biochem. J. 116: 693 (1970).
4. Farber, E. Studies on the molecular mechanisms of carcinogenesis. In: Homologies in Enzymes and Metabolic Pathways: Metabolic Alterations in Cancer, W.H. Whelan and J. Schultz, (Editors). North Holland Publishing Co., Amsterdam (1970).
5. Ryser, H.J-P. Chemical carcinogensis. New Eng. J. Med. 285: 721 (1971).
6. Magee, P.N. and J.M. Barnes. Carcinogenic nitroso compounds. Advances in Cancer Res. 10: 163 (1967).
7. Stekol, J.A. Biochemical basis for ethionine effects on tissues. Adv. Enzymol. 25: 369 (1963).
8. Farber, E. Ethionine carcinogenesis. Advances in Cancer Res. 7: 383 (1963).
9. Lawley, P.D. Effects of some chemical mutagens and carcinogens on nucleic acids. Prog. Nucleic Acid Res. Mol. Biol. 5: 89 (1966).
10. Farber, E. Carcinogenesis: cellular evolution as the unifying thread. Cancer Res., in press.
11. Lieberman, M.W., R.N. Baney, R.E. Lee, S. Sell and E. Farber. Studies on DNA repair in human lymphocytes treated with proximate carcinogens and alkylating agents. Cancer Res. 31: 1297 (1971).
12. Stich, H.F. and B.A. Laishes. DNA repair and chemical carcinogens. Pathobiology Annual, in press.
13. Cox, R., I. Damjanov, S. Abanobi and D.S.R. Sarma. A method for measuring DNA damage and repair in the liver *in vivo*. Cancer Res., in press.
14. Damjanov, I., R. Cox, D.S.R. Sarma and E. Farber. Patterns of damage and repair of liver deoxyribonucleic acid induced by carcinogenic methylating agents *in vivo*. Cancer Res., in press.
15. Haese, W.H., D.L. Smith and E. Bueding. Hycanthone-induced hepatic changes in mice infected with *Schisto-*

soma mansoni.   J. Pharmacol. Exp. Ther., in press.

16. Hanawalt, P.C.   Repair of genetic material in liver cells.   Endeavour 113: 83 (1972).
17. Painter, R.B.   Repair of DNA in mammalian cells. Current Topics Radiation Res. 7: 45 (1970).
18. Sarma, D.S.R., S. Rajalakshmi and E. Farber.   Interaction of chemical carcinogens with nucleic acids. In: Cancer: A Comprehensive Treatise, F.F. Becker (Editor).   Plenum Press, New York, in press.
19. Farber, E.   Hyperplastic liver nodules.   Methods Cancer Res. 7: 345 (1973).

HISTONE PHOSPHORYLATION AND THE CONTROL OF CELLULAR PROLIFERATION

Thaddeus W. Borun, Woon Ki Paik and Dawn Marks

Introduction

The data of many early studies of histone phosphorylation and especially histone f_1 phosphorylation were seen to be consistant with the hypothesis that this post-transcriptional modification was involved in processes leading to the selective activation and transcription of previously inactive genes in a number of different cellular systems (1-5). More recently, as techniques for the isolation and identification of phosphorylated histone polypeptides free of contaminating material (6-9) came to be widely employed (3,10-13) additional hypotheses concerning the function of histone f_1 and other histone phosphorylations have been suggested. Chalkley and his co-workers, after demonstrating a strong correlation between cellular proliferation and histone f_1 phosphorylation in a wide variety of systems (10,15-18), have emphasized the importance of the apparent relationship between the DNA replication occuring during cellular proliferation and histone f_1 phosphorylation (19). Dixon and co-workers, modifying an earlier hypothesis (20), have suggested that histone phosphate groups might facilitate a finishing interaction between DNA and histone molecules during chromosome replication in developing trout sperm cells (12). Speculations in this direction have recently been seriously complicated by the studies of Lake and Salzman (13), Bradbury *et al.* (30) and Gurley *et al.* (11) which emphasize the importance of a close relationship between the phosphorylation of histone f_1 and mitotic processes in synchronized Chinese hamster cells and in Physarum polycephalum.

For the past two years we have been examining the phosphorylation of histones during the Hela S-3 cell cycle as part of a larger systematic study of the relationship of

187

histone post-transcriptional modifications to the processes which control the concurrent synthesis of DNA and histones in this continuously dividing malignant cell. The results of the studies we shall discuss here suggest that there are at least two distinct kinds of Hela histone phosphorylation. The quantitatively most important of these modifications is a phosphorylation-dephosphorylation cycle which involves over 90% of the "old" and newly synthesized histone f_1 molecules. This phosphorylation cycle appears to be related to both S phase chromosome replication events and later mitotic phenomena but not increases in RNA synthesis or gene activation during the Hela S-3 cell cycle. After reviewing the experiments which support these conclusions we shall consider some of the possible implications of the histone f_1 phosphorylation cycle and its relationship to the processes which control proliferation in normal and transformed cells.

Methods

Purification of histone fractions by acrylamide gel electrophoresis

In many early studies of histone phosphorylation, the incorporation of ^{32}P into relatively crude histone fractions after various labeling periods was used as an index of histone phosphorylation (22,23). It soon became clear that lipids containing phosphorous, oligonucleotides and non-histone phosphoproteins all could have contaminated these preparations and lead to spurious conclusions concerning histone phosphorylation rates (6,10). Before beginning our own studies of Hela phosphorylation, we wished to determine whether the purification of acid-soluble nuclear extracts by electrophoresis toward the cathod in acrylamide gels containing urea and acetic acid was an effective means of removing ^{32}P labeled, non-histone contamination from labeled histone preparations. We therefore incubated early S phase Hela S-3 cells with ^{32}P orthophosphate for an hour, extracted the "histone" fraction from the nuclei with 0.25 N H_2SO_4 and resolved the component histone polypeptides by acrylamide gel electrophoresis according to the method of Panyim and Chalkley (21) as described in detail elsewhere (14). It can be seen

188

in Table 1 that pre-treatment of the crude nuclear extracts with a variety of lipid solvents has no effect on the amount of radioactivity eventually recovered from the ^{32}P incorporating peaks found in gels of the type shown in Figure 1. The most slowly migrating peak co-electrophoreses with histone f_1, the most rapidly migrating peak is associated with histone f_{2a1} while the middle peak could associated with either a slowly migrating form of histone f_{2a2} (18) or as would appear from the data itself, with histone f_{2b}. Because of this uncertainty we have referred to the central region of incorporation in the gel patterns as the $f_{2b}(f_{2a2})$ peak. Since pre-extraction of lipids has no effect on the radioactivity eventually found associated with the histone fractions in the gels we concluded that phospholipid contamination was not significant in histones purified solely by this kind of electrophoresis. The distribution of ^{32}P radioactivity in phosphorylated amino acids recovered from the histone f_1 region of the gels after extraction of the protein, hydrolysis and amino acid chromatography (14) is shown in Figure 2. About 88% of the amino acid radioactivity recovered after hydrolysis was found associated with phosphoserine region of the chromatogram. These results exclude the possibility of significant non-protein contamination co-electrophoresing with the histones on the gels. Since acidic or negatively charged non-histone phosphoproteins should migrate away from the cathode in this gel system, we concluded that we could accurately quantitate levels of ^{32}P incorporation into different histones and use such determinations as a valid index of histone phosphorylation levels. Similar electrophoretic techniques, evolved independently in other laboratories have since come to be accepted as more or less standard methods of estimating ^{32}P incorporation into histone phosphates (10-13).

Synchronization procedures

In a number of previous studies of histone phosphorylation in synchronized cells, the cell populations were a) "naturally" but poorly synchronized in regenerating rat liver (10), b) synchronized by isoleucine starvation, then refeeding (11), or c) were blocked in mitosis with colcemid, then released from the drug blockade (13,18). It is probable that none of these synchronizing techniques is

TABLE 1

Treatment of histone preparation with organic solvents to
remove contaminating phospholipids

"Crude" histone	Radioactivity found in (cpm)		
extract treatment	f_1	f_{2b}	f_{2a1}
None	443	201	97
Precipitated with ethanol at 4°C	496	208	99
Washed successively with ethanol, and with mixture of $CHCl_3$:ethanol:ether	482	250	88

One hundred μg of each histone sample were analyzed on
polyacrylamide gels containing 6 M urea which were electrophoresed for 12 hours at room temperature (1 mA/gel). Each
of the histone samples was obtained from 7.7×10^6 cells
(from an unsynchronized culture) labeled with 60 μC ^{32}P
for one hour.

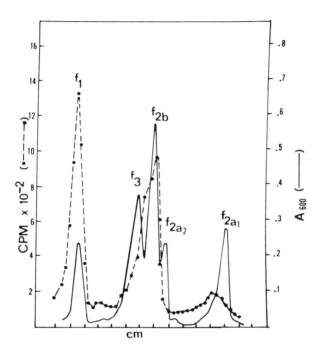

Fig. 1. ^{32}P *incorporation into histone fractions separated by polyacrylamide gel electrophoresis.* (o----o) ^{32} cpm. (————) Absorbance at 600 nanometers of the stained histone bands. A 25 cm gel containing 2 M urea was electrophoresed at 190 V for 26 hours. The histones were extracted from 3 x 10^6 cells which had been labeled for 30 min with 144 μCi ^{32}P in early S phase. Electrophoresis is from left to right (+ to -). Only the section of the gel containing the histone bands is shown. The lack of exact coincidence between the absorbance and the radioactivity may be due to a decrease in mobility experienced by the small population of molecules which are phosphorylated.

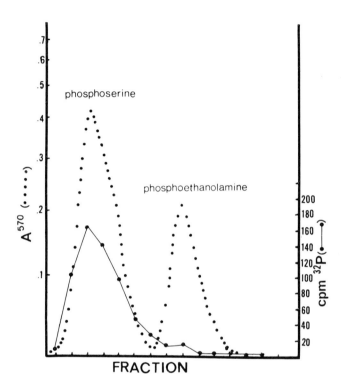

Fig. 2. *Recovery of radioactivity in f_1 histone fraction as ^{32}P phosphoserine.* The f_1 bands were cut from gels, hydrolyzed and the amino acids were separated by means of a Beckman automatic amino acid analyzer as described in the Experimental Procedures of reference 14. Of the 736 cmp placed on the column, 648 or (88%) were recovered in the phosphoserine fraction. (o————o), ^{32}P; (---------), A_{570}.

entirely satisfactory or gives as reliable an insight into
what is happening at all stages of the cell cycle as the
results obtained using cell populations synchronized by
selectively detaching cells in mitosis (24-26). For example, preliminary observations in our laboratory suggest
that colcemid treatment leads to the appearance of anomolous forms of histone f_1 phosphates and Lake (27) has
reported abnormal levels of histone phosphokinases in cells
during colcemid blockade. To reduce to a minimum the
possibility that our synchronization procedure was itself
influencing histone phosphorylation reactions we used only
cultures that had been synchronized by selective detachment
in mitosis. In Hela S-3 cells, mitosis lasts for about
one hour and is followed by a G_1 phase which is normally
about five hours long. DNA and histones are concurrently
synthesized during the S phase which follows G_1 and this
synthesis lasts for about 8-9 hours. G_2 follows S phase
beginning at about 15-16 hours after mitosis and lasts
until the cells have completed their 19-20 hour life cycle
and once again divide.

Results

*Estimates of histone phosphorylation and histone
phosphate turnover rates during the Hela S-3 cell cycle*

^{32}P Orthophosphate Incorporation Experiments

The amount of radioactivity incorporated into a phosphorylated histone after exposure of cells to medium con-
tainine ^{32}P orthophosphate is influenced by a complex set
of factors. Some of these factors include phosphate pool
size, amounts of histone polypeptides available for phosphorylation, histone kinase activity levels, histone phosphatase activity levels and histone phosphate exchange
reactions. The latter reactions could gradually replace
non-radioactive phosphates with labeled ones leading to
no net change in the amount of phosphorylated histone but
causing an increase in the specific activity of the histone
phosphate and complicating the interpretation of incorporation data. In the following experiments we used a combination of ^{32}P orthophosphate pulse-chase, continuous incorporation and pulse labeling to infer levels of histone

phosphorylation and determine histone phosphorylation turnover rates.

The accumulation of ^{32}P in histones during the Hela S-3 cell cycle

To estimate the net result of histone phosphorylation, dephosphorylation and phosphate exchange reactions we added ^{32}P orthophosphate to a culture of Hela S-3 cells at one hour after selective detachment in mitosis and incubated the cells in this radioactive medium for the rest of the cell cycle. At the times indicated in Figure 3 we removed cell samples, extracted the 0.25 NH_2SO_4 soluble nuclear fraction, resolved the component histones by electrophoresis on acrylamide gels and quantitated the histone mass and associated ^{32}P radioactivity as described in detail elsewhere (14). To emphasize changes in incorporation per unit mass of histone polypeptide we expressed the results of these determinations shown in Figure 3A as incorporation per arbitrary A_{600} units. In that Figure we have also compared histone specific activity changes with changes in the specific activity of DNA isolated from the same labeled cell samples at the indicated times. Histones f_{2a1} and $f_{2b}(f_{2a2})$ gradually increase in specific activity through G_1 and early S phase, then reach and maintain plateau values in G_2 which are about twice their average G_1 levels. Histone f_1 accumulated ^{32}P to much higher specific activities throughout the cell cycle, beginning in G_1 and continuing through G_2. By the end of the incorporation period the ratio $f_1:f_{2a1}:f_{2b}(f_{2a2})$ specific activities is about 14:2:1. Normalized increases in DNA and histone f_1 specific activities are shown in Figure 3B. It is evident that label accumulates in histone f_1 phosphate throughout G_1 prior to the initiation of DNA replication, then increases its rate of accumulation during S phase DNA replication until both DNA and histone f_1 specific activities reach plateaus in G_2. These data suggest that histone f_1 phosphorylation is qualitatively different and quantitatively more extensive than the phosphorylations of histones f_{2a1} and $f_{2b}(f_{2a2})$. Furthermore, it is apparent that "old" histones can be phosphorylated since ^{32}P is incorporated by the histones during G_1 prior to the synthesis of new polypeptides.

194

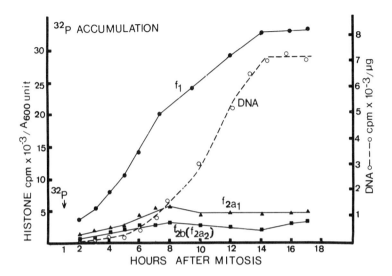

Figure 3A. *Accumulation of* [32]P-*label in histones of HeLa cells which were continuously exposed to* [32]P *throughout the cycle.* [32]P was added to the cultures one hr after mitosis. Aliquots were taken from the cultures at the times indicated, and histones were isolated by acid extraction and separated by electrophoresis on 6 M urea gels (1 mA/gel, 16 hrs). The absorbance of the stained histone bands was determined and the specific activity was calculated (cpm/A_{600} unit) after the amount of radioactivity in gel slices was measured. Data from two experiments were normalized and plotted together. In the first experiment cells were labeled (9 μCi ^{32}P/ml) in complete medium A (14). In the second experiment cells were labeled (14 μCi ^{32}P/ml) in Medium A containing 1/10 the normal amount of phosphate. (o———o), specific activity of histone f_1; (———), histone $f_{2b}(f_{2a2})$; Δ———Δ, histone f_{2a1}; 0-----0, specific activity of DNA determined as described in Experimental Procedure of 14.

32P ACCUMULATION

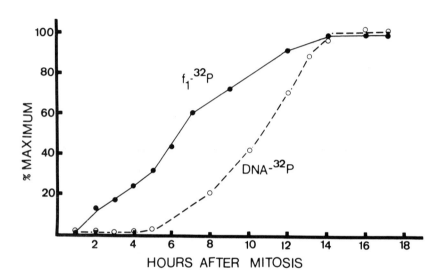

Fig. 3B. *Percent of maximum incorporation of* [32]P *into histone* f_1 *and DNA during continuous labeling of synchronized Hela cells.* (o————o), histone f_1; o—— ——o, DNA. Values are calculated from the data given in Figure 3A.

Histone phosphate turnover rate determinations

To determine how long phosphate groups remain associated with different histone polypeptides and to determine whether phosphate turnover rates are different in G_1 and S phase, we did the following pulse-chase experiments. One sample of a synchronized culture was incubated with ^{32}P for 60 minutes at one hour after mitosis (G_1), then the cells were harvested and resuspended and incubated in non-radioactive medium for up to six hours afterward. At the times indicated in Figures 4B and 4C cell samples were removed, histones were extracted and the radioactivity associated with different histones resolved by electrophoresis on acrylamide gels was determined as previously described (14). Another cell sample from the same synchronized culture was subjected to these procedures beginning at eight hours after mitosis (S phase). The pulse-labeling times in this experiment, relative to the rate of DNA replication in the cell samples are shown in Figure 4A. In Figure 4B it can be seen that the rate of incorporation of ^{32}P radioactivity into histone f_1 during the 60 minute pulse-labeling period increases about 10-fold as the cells proceed from G_1 into S phase. During that transition, the rate of ^{32}P incorporation into histones f_{2a1} and $f_{2b}(f_{2a2})$ also increased but only about 2-3-fold. When these data are normalized as shown in Figure 4C it is evident that although more label is incorporated and lost per unit time in S phase than in G_1, the percentage of the total previously incorporated histone phosphate radioactivity lost per unit chase time is very similar in both phases of the Hela S-3 cell cycle. Thus 10-15% of the ^{32}P radioactivity associated with histone f_1 and about 50% of the radioactivity associated with histones f_{2a1} and $f_{2b}(f_{2a2})$ is lost per hour in both G_1 and S phase. With the data presently available it is not possible to determine whether the loss of histone phosphate label is due to net dephosphorylation or only phosphate exchange reactions. However, these data do strongly reinforce the conclusion suggested in the preceeding section that the reactions affecting histone f_1 phosphate groups are different from those affecting histones f_{2a1} and $f_{2b}(f_{2a2})$.

197

The relationship of DNA and RNA synthesis to the rate of histone phosphorylation during the Hela S-3 cell cycle

To estimate how the rates of different histone phosphorylations vary in relation to DNA and RNA synthesis through the Hela cell cycle we pulse labeled cell samples with ^{32}P for 30 minutes at the times indicated in Figure 5. Labeled DNA, RNA and histones were isolated from each of the samples and the specific activities of thes macromolecules were determined as described in detail elsewhere (14). The apparent rates of histone f_{2a1} and $f_{2b}(f_{2a2})$ phosphorylation are rather low in G_1 then increase in early S phase leading to about a two-fold increase in the specific activities of these histones through the rest of S and G_2 (Figure 5A). These apparent rate increases closely parallel and are probably responsible for the increases in histone f_{2a1} and $f_{2b}(f_{2a2})$ phosphorylation do not parallel changes in the rates of DNA replication or RNA synthesis occuring during the Hela S-3 cell cycle. The phosphorylations of histones f_{2a1} and $f_{2b}(f_{2a2})$ thus do not appear to be obviously related to the increased RNA synthesis or "gene activation" which occurs during early G_1 in these cells.

In contrast to the behavior of histones f_{2a1} and $f_{2b}(f_{2a2})$ in this respect, changes in the apparent rate of histone f_1 phosphorylation do closely follow changes in the rate of DNA replication during G_1 and early S phase (Figure 5B). In this particular experiment, DNA replication, for unknown reasons, began about an hour earlier than is usually observed in these cells, increasing appreciably by about 4 hours after mitosis. In more typical experiments, such as the one shown in Figure 6, the rates of histone f_1 phosphorylation and DNA replication increased in parallel at about 5-6 hours after mitosis as the cells passed from G_1 into S phase. The close linkage of DNA synthesis and histone f_1 phosphorylation rates in G_1 and early S phase does not persist into late S and G_2. It can be seen in Figure 5B that at 16 hours after mitosis when the rate of DNA replication has declined to 30% of its maximum value the apparent rate of histone f_1 phosphorylation is still at 60% of its maximum level. We feel that these and other data to be presented later suggest that the decline in the rate of histone f_1 phosphorylation observed in the latter portions of the cell cycle is more closely correlated with an

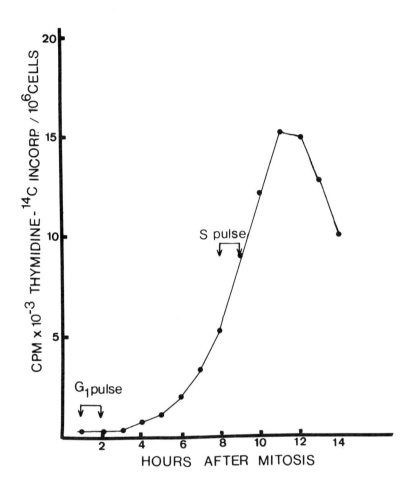

Fig. 4A. *The incorporation of thymidine 2 ^{14}C into 5% TCA precipitable form into 1 x 10^6 cells during g_1 and early S phase pulsed with 2 μC of isotope in 2 ml of complete medium for 30 minutes as described in the Experimental Procedures of 14.*

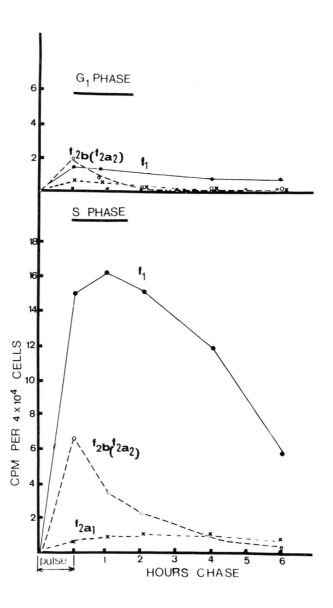

Fig. 4B. *The rate of dephosphorylation of pulse-labeled Hela histones.* At one hr after mitosis (G_1) 2 x 10^8 synchronized Hela S-3 cells were pulsed with 4.3 mC ^{32}P for one hr in medium A containing 1/10 normal phosphate. The cells were then sedimented and resuspended at 5 x 10^5 cells/ml in complete medium A containing no ^{32}P. Samples of 4 x 10^7 cells were taken at the indicated times, the extracted histone were electrophoresed (2 M urea gels, 26 hrs, 190 V), and the amount of radioactivity remaining in the histone fractions was determined. 2 x 10^8 synchronized Hela S-3 cells were also pulsed during S (8 hr after mitosis) for one hr with 4.3 mC ^{32}P. After resuspension to a concentration of 5 x 10^5 cells/ml samples of 4 x 10^7 cells were taken for histone isolation and electrophoresis as described above and in the Experimental Procedure of 14. Histones from 4 x 10^6 cells were electrophoresed on each gel following the G_1 pulse, while 2 x 10^6 cells were used following the S pulse (o———o), f_1 histone; (o------o), f_{2b} (f_{2a2}); (x-----x), f_{2a1}.

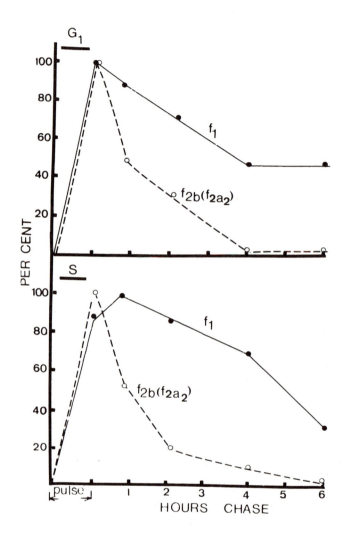

Fig. 4C. *The percent of ^{32}P remaining in histone fractions f_1 and f_{2b} (f_{2a2}) after a pulse during G_1 or S as described in the legend of figure 4B.*

202

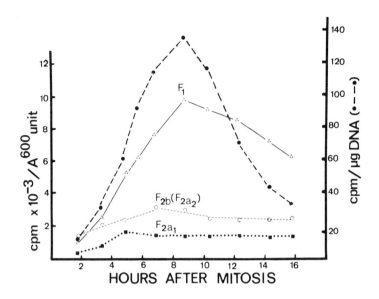

Fig. 5A. *Specific activity of Hela histone fractions after*
^{32}P *pulses at various times during the cell cycle.* Fifty
ml aliquots were taken at the indicated times for a culture
containing 6.2×10^5 synchronized cells/ml. The aliquot
was sedimented, resuspended for one-half hr in 10 ml
medium A containing one-tenth the normal amount of phosphate and 730 μC ^{32}P, and the histones were isolated. The
histones (corresponding to 3.4×10^6 cells/gel) were electrophoresed (6 M urea, 16 hrs, 1 mA/gel). The absorbance
at 600 nanometers of the stained histone bands was determined and the specific activity was calculated (cpm/A_{600}
unit) after the amount of radioactivity in gel slices was
determined. The specific activity of DNA was determined
as described under Materials and Methods of 14. (Δ———Δ),
histone f_1; o------o, f_{2b} (f_{2a2}); -----, f_{2a1}; and o———o,
DNA.

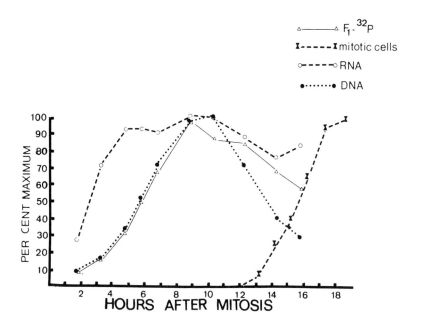

Fig. 5B. *The temporal relationship of f_1 histone phosphorylation, nucleic acid synthesis and percent cells accumulating in metaphase after colcamide treatment during HeLa cell cycle.* Aliquots of a synchronized culture were pulsed with ^{32}P as described in Figure 5A. The histones were isolated, electrophoresed and the amount of radioactivity in histone f_1 was determined by counting gel slices. DNA and RNA were isolated from nuclear pellets remaining after histone extraction, and separated as described in Experimental Procedures of reference 14. Aliquots were counted to determine the extent of ^{32}P incorporation, and the results are presented as percent of maximum incorporation. Colcamide was added to a concentration of .05 µl/ml to a part of the culture at 12 hours after mitosis and the percent of cells accumulating in metaphase was determined by phase contract microscopy. (X-----X), metaphase cells; Δ———Δ, f_1 histone; o———o, DNA; o-----o, RNA.

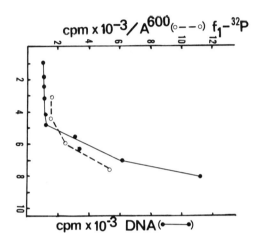

Fig. 6. *The first portion of the experiment described in Figures 5A and 5B was repeated to demonstrate the low rates of f_1 phosphorylation and DNA replication which usually occur throughout G_1.* (o———o) Rate of DNA replication; o-----o, specific activity of f_1 phosphorylation measured by ^{32}P pulses for 30 minutes.

increase in the number of cells entering and then passing through mitosis (Figure 5B) than with declines in the rate of DNA replication. It can also be seen in Figure 5B that histone f_1 phosphorylation rate increases or decreases are not temporally correlated with G_1 "gene activation" or increases in RNA synthesis rates in the Hela cell.

The effect of cytosine arabinoside on histone phosphorylation in G_1 and S phase

To determine if there was an obligatory coupling between increased histone f_1 phosphorylation rates and DNA replication we pulse-labeled control and cytosine arabinoside treated cells with ^{32}P for 30 minutes at the times in G_1 and S phase shown in Figure 7A. The histones were extracted from the cells and analyzed on acrylamide gels as described elsewhere (14). It can be seen in Figure 7B that cytosine arabinoside at a concentration (40 µg/ml) which inhibits DNA replication and histone synthesis (28, 29) in these cells has no effect on histone f_{2a1} and f_{2b} (f_{2a2}) phosphorylation rates in either G_1 or S phase. The drug inhibits about 50% of the S phase histone f_1 phosphorylation but has no effects on the low G_1 levels of incorporation observed in this fraction.

All of the data presented so far imply a clear distinction between the phosphorylations affecting histone f_{2a1} and f_{2b}(f_{2a2}) and those which affect histone f_1 molecules. The specific activity of histone f_1 during S phase and G_2 is much higher than that observed in the other histone fractions in accumulation, pulse-chase and in pulse labeling experiments. The turnover rate of histone f_1 phosphate groups is 3-4 times slower than the turnover of histone f_{2a1} and f_{2b}(f_{2a2}) phosphates. Finally the phosphorylations of histones f_{2a1} and f_{2b}(f_{2a2}) do not appear to be directly coupled to DNA replication in any obvious way although they may be related in some fashion to chromosomal replication and processing since they do seem to increase about 2-3-fold as the cells pass through S and G_2 while proceeding towards mitosis. Histone f_1 phosphorylation on the other hand does seem to have some sort of direct couple with DNA replication in G_1 and early S phase since its rate increases about 10-fold as the cells pass from the one phase to the next. Furthermore, about half of the phosphate incorporation into histone f_1 in S phase can be in-

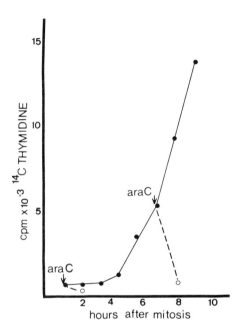

Fig. 7A. *The effect of cytosine arabinoside on DNA synthesis during G_1 and early S phases of the Hela cell cycle.*
Two ml aliquots of a synchronized cell culture (4.3×10^5
cells/ml) were taken at the indicated times and pulsed with
0.2 µC of thymidine-^{14}C for 30 min at 37°. The amount of
radioactivity incorporated into 5% TCA precipitable material was used as an index of DNA synthesis. In G_1 and S,
aliquots were treated for one hr with 40 µg of cytosine
arabinoside/ml prior to and during the thymidine pulse.
o———o, control cells. o-----o, cells after cytosine
arabinoside treatment.

207

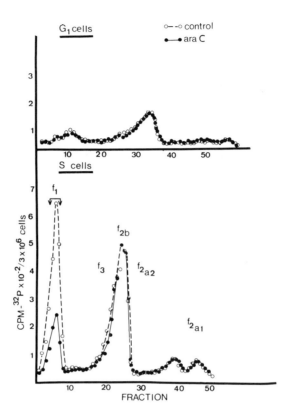

Fig. 7B. *The effect of cytosine arabinoside on the phosphorylation of various histone fractions during G_1 and S.*
At one hr (G_1) and 7 hrs (S) after mitosis, cytosine arabinoside (40 μg/ml of cells) was added to aliquots of cells from the culture described in Fig. 7A. One hr later control and cytosine arabinoside-treated cells were pulsed for 30 min with ^{32}P (50 μC/ml x 10^6 cells). Histones were then isolated and electrophoresed (2 M urea, 26 hrs, 190 V). The amount of radioactivity in each histone was determined by counting gel slices. o-----o, control cells; o———o, cells treated with cytosine arabinoside.

hibited by inhibiting DNA replication. At this point in
time the function or functions of histone f_{2a1} and f_{2b}
(f_{2a2}) are not known and will probably remain unknown until
methods are developed for determining how the masses of
these phosphorylated histone species change through the
cell cycle, and clear correlations between the mass changes
and various cell cycle events can be established. Recently
Chalkley and his associates (10) reported a technique which
allows a direct determination of the mass of the different
phosphorylated and non-phosphorylated forms of histone f_1
by high resolution acrylamide gel electrophoresis. In
the following experiments we used this technique to study
changes in different histone f_1 species through the Hela
cell cycle.

*Resolution and quantitation of different forms of
histone f_1 during the Hela S-3 cell cycle*

To determine how the amounts of different phosphorylated and unphosphorylated forms of histone f_1 changed through
the Hela cell cycle, we isolated histones from control and
cytosine arabinoside treated synchronized cells at the times
after mitosis indicated in Figure 8A and analyzed them using the high resolution acrylamide gel electrophoresis
technique described by Balhorn *et al*. (10). It can be seen
in Figures 8B and 8C that histone f_1 polypeptides can be
resolved into three distinct forms in the Hela cell. Form
I is probably not phosphorylated since it does not incorporate ^{32}P radioactivity and its migration rate is unaffected by digestion with alkaline phosphatase. Forms II
and III do incorporate ^{32}P and Form III is caused to migrate more quickly by alkaline phosphatase digestion. The
migration of the two putative phosphorylated forms are such
that it is probable that histone f_1 Form II is monophos-
phorylated and Form III is diphosphorylated. The gel patterns of stained f_1 histones from cells at different times
are shown in Figure 9A. It is evident that the Form III or
putative histone f_1 diphosphate begins accumulating as the
cells enter S phase and begin synthesizing DNA and histone
molecules. This accumulation continues through S into G_2
and mitosis. By the end of G_2, well after the DNA replication rate has declined to low levels, over 90% of the histone f_1 polypeptides remain in the mono- or di-phosphoryla-
ted forms. After mitosis histone f_1 Form III is almost

completely degraded during early G_1 and is not reformed until S phase and the phosphorylation cycle simultaneously begin once again. If the cells are treated with cytosine arabenoside (ara C) in G_1 so that DNA replication does not begin, the formation of histone f_1, Form III commences at its usual time in S phase (Figure 9B), and previously synthesized of "old" histone f_1 molecules are phosphorylated. It can also be seen in the same Figure that if DNA replication is prematurely terminated in S phase by ara C treatment the accumulation of Form III continues but at a reduced rate, suggesting that newly synthesized histone f_1 molecules are phosphorylated as well as "old" molecules.

These quantitations give a good perspective for interpreting the ^{32}P incorporation data in the preceeding sections. First, it is clear that the G_1 accumulation of ^{32}P in histone f_1 prior to the initiation of DNA replication does not reflect the net accumulation of histone f_1 phosphates since the more highly phosphorylated Form III is degraded to the less phosphorylated Form II and the unphosphorylated Form I during G_1 of the Hela cell cycle. This G_1 accumulation, also noted by Shepherd *et al.* (22) in Chinese hamster cells, may reflect the results of exchange reactions which replace non-radioactive Form II phosphates with labeled ones during the accumulation period. Second, the increased rate of histone f_1 phosphorylation observed as the cells pass from G_1 into S and G_2 probably reflects the extensive net accumulation of histone f_1 Form III at those times. Third, the lack of strict coupling of DNA replication rates in G_2 with the retention of Form III molecules in the cell implies that histone f_1 phosphorylation are probably not only related to DNA polymerization reactions but may also be involved in the processes which move chromosomes about relative to one another as they are replicated and then prepared for condensation and separation during mitosis. The present data therefore may be interpreted as suggesting that phosphorylated histone f_1 molecules may be involved in a replication and chromosome processing complex which is used during S, G_2 and mitosis but is rapidly degraded as the cells pass out of mitosis into G_1.

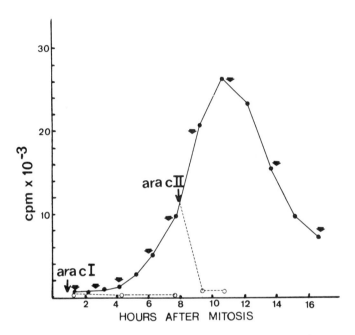

Fig. 8A. *The effect of cytosine arabinoside on DNA synthesis when administered at 1 to 7 hrs after mitosis.* o————o, control cells, o-----o, cytosine arabinoside treated cells. Arrows indicate points at which samples of 4×10^7 cells were removed for histone extraction as described in the Experimental Procedure of reference 14.

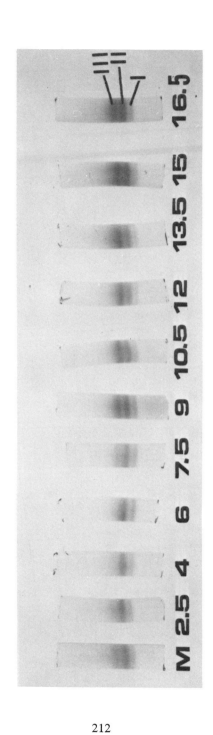

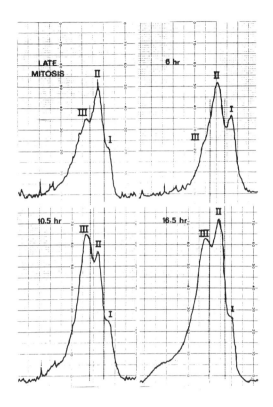

Fig. 8B and 8C. *The three forms of histone f_1 resolved on high resolution polyacrylamide gels.* The stained gels (25 cm in length, containing 25 M urea, run at 200 V for 68.5 hrs at 4°) were aligned, and the f_1 regions were cut out, photographed and scanned. Forms I, II and III are indicated as well as the time (in hours after mitosis) at which the histones were isolated. B) Photographs of the f_1 region. Electrophoresis is from top to bottom. C) Patterns of the absorbance at 600 nanometers of the f_1 region of four of the gels shown in B. Electrophoresis is from left to right.

213

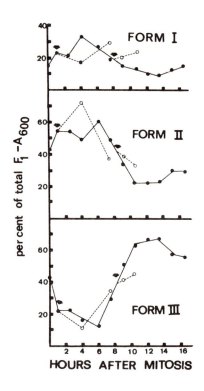

Fig. 9. *The percent of total histone f_1 found during the cell cycle under the areas designated Form I, II or III described in Fig. 7.* o———o, control; 0-----0, cytosine arabinoside treated. The arrows indicate the time at which cytosol arabinoside was added to a portion of the culture. The inhibitor was present from this time until the histones were isolated from the treated samples.

Summary and Conclusion

It has been suggested that histone phosphorylation was related to processes which control a) selective RNA transcription (1-5), b) histone transport from cytoplasm to nucleus (19,31), c) DNA replication (10,12,15-18) and d) mitosis (11,13,30). The data discussed here and reported in detail elsewhere (14) strongly support a relationship between f_1 phosphorylation, DNA replication and mitosis in continuously proliferating malignant Hela S-3 cells. The histone phosphorylations observed in this cell type do not appear to be related to histone transport nor do they exhibit any obvious relationship to selective RNA transcription processes. Hela histone phosphorylations are complex phenomena, in that the phosphorylations affecting histones f_{2a1} and $f_{2b}(f_{2a2})$ appear to be quite different from those affecting histone f_1 polypeptides. Because it is not yet possible to accurately quantitate changes in the mass of histone f_{2a1} and $f_{2b}(f_{2a2})$ phosphates through the cell cycle the function of those phosphorylations remain unknown. However a reasonable hypothesis concerning the function of histone f_1 phosphorylation can be proposed and we would like to conclude with a discussion of that hypothesis.

The present data (14) and the data of many previous studies (10-13,15-19,30) are consistent with the idea that certain phosphorylated forms of histone f_1 molecules are part of an active chromosomal replication and pre-mitotic processing complex which is present in proliferating cells from the beginning of S phase through G_2 and mitosis. The degradation of histone f_1 Form III (putative diphosphorylated f_1 molecules) in early G_1, the nearly complete absence of analogous phosphorylated histone f_1 molecules in non-proliferating G_0 cells (10,16) suggest that histone f_1 molecules which are not sufficiently phosphorylated are inactive or incapable of participating in such a replication and processing complex. If the preceeding premises are true then control of histone f_1 phosphorylation may be the mechanism by which chromosomal replication and cellular proliferation are controlled. Cells which stop proliferating in G_0 of the cell cycle may be stopped there because they cannot initiate replication of their chromosomes. The present hypothesis suggests that they may not be able to replicate their chromosomes because they are for some reason unable to phosphorylate histone f_1 to the necessary level and thereby initiate the replication reactions. A number of lines of evidence are consistent with this hypothesis which in contrast to early hypotheses (12,13,14,30) stresses equally the relationship of histone f_1 phosphorylation to both DNA replication and mitosis.

1. Many physical and metabolic characteristics distinguish histone f_1 from the other four principle histone molecules (for a review of many of these properties see reference 32). Perhaps the most notable of these distinguishing characteristics include its larger size, extensive tissue and species variability, the ease with which it can be extracted from chromatin by ionic reagents and its apparent capacity to cross link DNA helices (32-34).

2. There are enough histone f_1 molecules in the cell and on chromosomes and enough of these molecules are phosphorylated during the cell cycle to be able to carry out the proposed control function (14,32). There are probably not enough molecules of other non-histone chromosomal proteins available to carry out identical control functions throughout the total genome (1,35). In the Hela S-3 cell, the acid soluble nuclear fraction comprises about 5% of the total cell protein and of that fraction at least 10-15% is histone f_1. This histone is thus almost 1% of the total cell's protein and perhaps as much as 5-10% of the protein in the nucleus.

3. Mirsky and his co-workers (36,37) have reported that histone f_1 more effectively blocks accessibility of chromatin to DNAase and DNA polymerase than any other histone fraction and that phosphorylation of histone f_1 appreciably reduces that blocking ability. Conversely, removal of histone f_1 or its phosphorylation leads to increased rates of replication reactions.

4. Histone f_1 phosphorylation has been shown to be affected by phosphokinase and phosphatase reactions which in turn are influenced by cellular levels of cyclic AMP (2,3,38,39). In light of the growing number of reports of a relationship between cellular proliferation and cyclic AMP levels in normal and transformed cells (40-43), histone f_1 phosphorylation becomes a very attractive candidate for the mechanism which controls DNA replication and thus proliferation (19) by mediating between cell surface stimuli (to start and stop proliferating) and the chromosomes. The present hypothesis concerning the control of cellular proliferation suggests the following relation-

ships.

A. Stimulation to proliferate or remain quiescent causes cell surface mediated reactions which lead to changes in intracellular cyclic nucleotide concentrations.

B. Changes in cyclic nucleotide concentrations lead to the increased activity of intranuclear histone f_1 kinases or decrease the activity of histone f_1 phosphatases leading to a net increase in histone f_1 diphosphate in the Hela cell or it analogues in other cellular systems.

C. Increased histone f_1 phosphorylation releases an exhibitory cross linkage of DNA helices, facilitating the activity of DNA replicating enzymes, perhaps by allowing access of DNAase molecules to specific nicking initiation points which then are points of entry of DNA polymerase molecules.

D. The histone f_1 phosphate would act not only in facilitating replication processes but may also act as part of a chromosomal complex in the nucleus which sorts out replicated chromosomal segments and prepares replicated chromosomes for mitotic condensations. Obviously much work is needed before this hypothesis can be proven or disproven and we are now in the process of examining various aspects of the hypothesis in the Hela S-3 and other cell types.

Presented by Thaddeus W. Borun from the Fels Research Institute and Department of Biochemistry, Temple University School of Medicine, Philadephia, Pennsylvania. The authors would like to recognize the excellent technical assistance of Barbara Keller and Alice Lu. Supported by grants from the National Institutes of Health, AM-09603, CA-10439, 12226, 11463, 1, PO1-HD 05874 and AM-18843-01.

References

1. Kleinsmith, L.J., V.G. Allfrey and A.E. Mirsky. Proc. Nat. Acad. Sci. USA 55: 1182 (1966).
2. Langan, T.A. Science 162: 579 (1968).
3. Langan, T.A. Proc. Nat. Acad. Sci. USA 64: 1276 (1969).
4. Stevely, W.S. and L.A. Stocken. Biochem. J. 110: 187 (1968).

5. Ord, M.A. and L.A. Stocken. Biochem. J. 107: 403 (1968).
6. Shephard, G.R., B.J. Noland and C.N. Roberts. Biochim. Biophys. Acta. 199: 265 (1970).
7. Hnilica, L.S. and L.C. Bess. Anal. Biochem. 12: 421 (1965).
8. Johns, E.W. Biochem. J. 92: 55 (1964).
9. Fambrough, D.M. and J. Bonner. J. Biol. Chem. 243: 4434 (1968).
10. Balhorn, R., W.O. Rieke and R. Chalkley. Biochem. 10: 3952 (1971).
11. Gurley, L.R., R.A. Walters and R.A. Tobey. Biochem. Biophys. Res. Commun. 50: 744 (1973).
12. Louie, A.J, M.T. Lung and G.H. Dixon. J. Biol. Chem. 248: 3335 (1973).
13. Lake, R.S. and N.P. Salzman. Biochem. 11: 4817 (1972).
14. Marks, D., W.-K. Paik and T.W. Borun. J. Biol. Chem. 235: 5660 (1973).
15. Sherod, D., G. Johnson and R. Chalkley. Biochem. 9: 4611 (1970).
16. Balhorn, R., R. Chalkley and D. Granner. Biochem. 11: 1094 (1972).
17. Balhorn, R., M. Balhorn, H.P. Morris and R. Chalkley. Cancer Res. 32: 1775 (1972).
18. Balhorn, R., J. Bordwell, L. Sellers, D. Granner and R. Chalkley. Biochem. Biophys. Res. Commun. 46: 1326 (1972).
19. Oliver, D., R. Balhorn, D. Granner and R. Chalkley. Biochem. 11: 3921 (1972).
20. Surrey, M.T. and G.H. Dixon. Proc. Nat. Acad Sci USA 67: 1616 (1970).
21. Panyim, S. and R. Chalkley. Arch. Biochem. Biophys. 130: 337 (1969).
22. Shepherd, G.R., B.J. Noland and J.M. Hardin. Arch. Biochem. Biophys. 142: 299 (1971).
23. Ord, M.C. and L.A. Stocken. Biochem. J. 112: 81 (1969).
24. Terasina, T. and L.J. Tolmach. Exp. Cell Res. 30: 344 (1963).
25. Robbins, E. and P. Marcus. Science 44: 1152 (1964).
26. Stein, G.S. and T.W. Borun. J. Cell Biol. 52: 792 (1972).
27. Lake, R.S. Nature New Biol. 242: 145 (1973).

28. Borun, T.W., M.D. Scharff and E. Robbins. Proc. Nat. Acad. Sci. USA 58: 1977 (1967).
29. Stein, G. and T.W. Borun. J. Cell. Biol. 52: 292 (1972).
30. Bradley, E.M., R.J. Inglis, H.R. Matthews and N. Sarner. Europ. J. Biochem. 33: 131 (1973).
31. Gurley, L.R., R.A. Walters and M.D. Enger. Biochem. Biophys. Res. Commun. 40: 428 (1970).
32. Hnilica, L.S. The Structure and Biological Functions of Histones, CRC Press (1973) Cleveland, Ohio, pp. 16-20, 84-88.
33. Cohen, L.H. and B.V. Gotchel. J. Biol. Chem. 246: 1841 (1971).
34. Simpson, R.T. Biochemistry 11: 2003 (1973).
35. Elgin, S.C.R. and J. Bonner. Biochemistry 22: 4440 (1970).
36. Mirsky, A.E., B. Silverman and N.C. Panda. Proc. Nat. Acad. Sci. USA 69: 3243 (1972).
37. Mirsky, A.E. and B. Silverman. Proc. Nat. Acad. Sci. USA 70: 1973 (1973).
38. Murray, A.W., M. Froscio and B.E. Kemp. Biochem. J. 129: 995 (1972).
39. Cross, M.E. and M.G. Ord. Biochem. J. 124: 241 (1971).
40. Whitfield, J.R., R.H. Rixon, J.P. McManus and S.D. Balk. In vitro 8: 257 (1973).
41. Otten, J., G.S. Johnson and I. Pastan. Biochem. Biophys. Res. Commun. 44: 1192 (1971).
42. Willingham, M.C., G.S. Johnson and I. Pastan. Biochem. Biophys. Res. Commun. 48: 743 (1972).
43. Sheppard, J.R. Proc. Nat. Acad. Sci. USA 68: 1316 (1971).

SUBJECT INDEX